Rehabilitation Strategies
for Sensorineural Hearing Loss

Proceedings of
The Second Symposium on the Application of
Signal Processing Concepts to Hearing Aids
Pennsylvania State University
University Park, Pennsylvania
March 23–24, 1979

GRUNE & STRATTON RAPID MANUSCRIPT REPRODUCTION

Rehabilitation Strategies for Sensorineural Hearing Loss

Edited by

Paul Yanick, Jr., M.A., C.C.C.A.
Adjunct Assistant Professor
Department of Electronic Engineering
Monmouth College
West Long Branch, N.J.

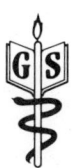

GRUNE & STRATTON
A Subsidiary of Harcourt Brace Jovanovich, Publishers
NEW YORK   LONDON   TORONTO   SYDNEY   SAN FRANCISCO

© 1979 by Grune & Stratton, Inc.
All rights reserved. No part of this publication
may be reproduced or transmitted in any form or
by any means, electronic or mechanical, including
photocopy, recording, or any information storage
and retrieval system, without permission in writing
from the publisher.

Grune & Stratton, Inc.
111 Fifth Avenue
New York, New York 10003

Distributed in the United Kingdom by
Academic Press, Inc. (London) Ltd.
24/28 Oval Road, London NW1

Library of Congress Catalog Number 79-3282
International Standard Book Number 0-8089-1215-1

Printed in the United States of America

To Mariská

CONTENTS

Preface ix

Contributors xi

Chapter 1
The Influence and Role of Otolaryngology in the Hearing
Rehabilitation Process   1
  Lindsay L. Pratt, M.D.

Chapter 2
New Concepts in Signal Processing and Hearing Rehabilitation   13
  Paul Yanick, Jr., M.A.

Chapter 3
Electrostimulation of the Cochlea: A Brief History   33
  James Martin, Ph.D.

Chapter 4
Real-Ear Measures of Hearing Aid Performance   75
  Geary A. McCandless, Ph.D.

Chapter 5
The Non-Universal Binaural Hearing Advantage   89
  Bruce Siegenthaler, Ph.D.

Chapter 6
The Otomandibular Syndrome   99
  Ira M. Klemons, D.D.S.

Chapter 7
Digital Processing Techniques in Speech Discrimination Testing
(Critical Band Measurements for Use in Hearing Aid Testing)   109
  Gordon R. Bienvenue, Ph.D. and Paul L. Michael, Ph.D.

Chapter 8
Digital Approaches to Auditory Training   129
  Harris Drucker, Ph.D.

Chapter 9
Post-Fitting Counseling of the Hearing Impaired Listener 145
   Steven W. Vargo, Ph.D.

Chapter 10
Audibility and Intelligibility of Speech for Listeners with
Sensorineural Hearing Loss 159
   Margaret W. Skinner, Ph.D.

Chapter 11
Summary of the Proceedings of the Symposium on the Application
of Signal Processing Concepts to Hearing Aids 185
   Joseph P. Millin, Ph.D.

Chapter 12
Panel Discussion: Hearing Aid Selection, Fitting, and Post-Fitting
Procedures 191
   Joseph P. Millin, Ph.D., Moderator

Chapter 13
Panel Discussion: Cochlear Electrostimulation 209
   Lindsay L. Pratt, M.D., Moderator

PREFACE

This book is dedicated to helping the millions of hearing aid wearers who, because of inaccurate fitting methods and inadequate counseling activities, are deprived of free and easy communication.

The volume's all-inclusive, idealistic goal is the emphasis of change. The changes that may be effectuated as a result of this symposium are probably small but because of the anatomy of any change, they require an abundance of resolve. There is a general tendency to resist change, though I hope the excitement of adding new dimensions to our professional practice will motivate others to overcome this resistance.

This volume also emphasizes the importance of the individual; that is, both the natural and common sense capacity that we can utilize to gain a better understanding of human communication and, more precisely, the consideration of the individual patient's feelings about, reactions to, and interpretation of compensatory amplification.

There is no doubt that some hearing aid problems are of an engineering nature, but most of them are a result of the misuse and abuse of electroacoustic amplification on an individual ear. For this reason, the book has been organized to stress the practical application of the relevant clinical and research papers presented at The Second Symposium on the Application of Signal Processing Concepts to Hearing Aids.

Since the audience consisted of hearing aid specialists, audiologists, and engineers, this symposium gave us an opportunity to join forces to solve many of the complex problems we face when we fit a hearing aid on a person with sensorineural hearing loss. This combined effort helped increase our understanding of how to apply the electroacoustic hearing aid to the sensorineural ear, which has undoubtedly benefited the hard of hearing people with whom we have come in contact since leaving this meeting. In addition, it has given us the satisfaction of knowing that a fuller professional service is being rendered.

This meeting would not have been possible without the support of Penn State University's Conference Center, the Department of Speech Pathology and Audiology, Mr. Kent Addis, and Dr. Bruce Seigenthaler. I would like to extend my sincere thanks to them and to all of the faculty members for the time and effort that they have so graciously given to make this symposium and the resulting text a complete and successful endeavor.

Finally, I would like to extend my sincere thanks to the contributors to this book for their fine work and to Janet Mednick for her invaluable help in preparing the manuscript.

PAUL YANICK, JR., M.A.

CONTRIBUTORS

Gordon R. Bienvenue, Ph.D.   Environmental Acoustics Lab
Pennsylvania State University
University Park, Pennsylvania

Harris Drucker, Ph.D.   Department of Electronic Engineering
Monmouth College
West Long Branch, New Jersey

Ira M. Klemons, D.D.S.   Director, Family Dental Center
Woodbridge, New Jersey

James Martin, Ph.D.   Department of Psychology
Pennsylvania State University
University Park, Pennsylvania

Geary A. McCandless, Ph.D.   Department of Speech and Hearing
University of Utah
Salt Lake City, Utah

Paul L. Michael, Ph.D.   Environmental Acoustics Lab
Pennsylvania State University
University Park, Pennsylvania

Joseph P. Millin, Ph.D.   School of Speech
Kent State University
Kent, Ohio

David P. Pascoe, Ph.D.   Central Institute for the Deaf
St. Louis, Missouri

Lindsay L. Pratt, M.D.   Department of Otolaryngology
Cooper Medical Center
Camden, New Jersey

Bruce Siegenthaler, Ph.D.   Department of Speech Pathology and Audiology
Pennsylvania State University
University Park, Pennsylvania

Margaret W. Skinner, Ph.D.   Central Institute for the Deaf
St. Louis, Missouri

Gerald A. Studebaker, Ph.D.   Program in Speech and Hearing Sciences
City University of New York
New York, New York

Steven W. Vargo, Ph.D.   Division of Otorhinolaryngology
Milton S. Hershey Medical Center
Hershey, Pennsylvania

Paul Yanick, Jr., M.A.   Department of Electronic Engineering
Monmouth College
West Long Branch, New Jersey

Rehabilitation Strategies
for Sensorineural Hearing Loss

Chapter 1

The Influence and Role of Otolaryngology in the Hearing Rehabilitation Process

Lindsay L. Pratt, M.D.

Hearing rehabilitation involves the mixture of medicine, hearing testing and assisting a patient in the psychological adjustment to the amplification they receive.

The role of the physician is only to establish the presence or absence of any medical diseases within the auditory system prior to the purchase of a hearing aid. The purpose of the physician is not to establish a patient's candidacy for a hearing aid.

The physician should be an otolaryngologist, knowledgeable in diseases of the ear, whose goal is to establish the medical parameters of an individual's hearing loss, offer appropriate treatment recommendations, and recruit the best qualified professionals to assist in the delivery of that treatment. In hearing aid dispensing, the physician should be qualified to identify the medical cause of the hearing loss; to provide qualified personnel to assist the hearing handicapped individual in their psychological adaptation to the amplification; to recommend the appropriate amplification, evaluation, and hearing aid selection and application at an appropriate cost; and to assure that the individual receives service necessary to support the hearing aid.

There is generalized agreement that an otolaryngologist, knowledgeable in diseases of the ear, is the only hearing health care professional with the medical background necessary to perform an appropriate medical examination of a hearing handicapped individual. Accordingly, the otolaryngologist is the best qualified physician to introduce a hearing handicapped individual into the auditory rehabilitation process.

But what about the word "physician" that appears in the legislation? A great deal of discussion has been raised concerning the use of the word "physician" rather than otolaryngologist.

The word "physician" is used in legislation because the word "otolaryngologist" is professionally restrictive and is prohibited by FTC regulations, as well as being incompatible with Justice Department anti-trust laws. The most qualifying statement permissable in legislation is "physician, preferably one knowledgeable in diseases of the ear".

A second criticism frequently expressed regarding hearing aid legislation is the use of the waiver. If the medical examination is essential to protect the patient's best medical interests prior to the purchase of a hearing aid, why is a waiver permitted?

In our form of government, it is impossible to mandate that individuals have a physical examination against their wishes. Accordingly, legislation can only recommend that an examination be provided the individual prior to the purchase of a hearing aid, and it requires the examiner to state that an individual's medical interests may be in jeopardy by not having the medical examination prior to the purchase of a hearing aid.

A frequent challenge to the role of the physician in hearing aid dispensing is the need for the medical examination prior to the purchase of a hearing aid. What does a medical examination contribute to a hearing aid selection?

As repeatedly stated, a medical examination contributes nothing to the hearing aid selection. The intent of the medical examination is only to assure that an individual's best medical interests are protected prior to the purchase of a hearing aid.

During the presentation of testimony before investigative committes, abuses within the hearing aid dispensing system were placed under three categories, as follows:

1. Hearing aids were placed upon individuals who were able to derive questionable benefit from the amplification.
2. Hearing aids were placed upon individuals at unreasonably high costs.
3. Hearing aids were placed upon individuals who had medical problems and should have had medical treatment prior to the application of the hearing aid.

The investigative committees were unable to find any common ground to propose legislation that could protect an individual from receiving an inappropriate hearing aid. Why?

The existing hearing aid evaluation and selection procedures possess no scientific credibility, are incapable of demanding accountability from tester, dispenser or manufacturer, possess no test-retest, different tester, or different dialect reliability.

The existing evaluation and selection procedures depend upon the subjective selection of a hearing aid by the examiner and the measurement of the hearing handicapped individual's response to the amplification provided by the subjectively selected hearing aid. Measureable objective standards do not exist and legislation is impossible without such objective standards.

As the tendency grows toward the use of frequency by frequency measurements as the method of recommending hearing aid amplification, the credibility of the evaluation systems will improve and legislative potential will then exist.

Presently there are no recommended hearing aid testing procedures capable of establishing a patient's candidacy for, benefit from, satisfaction with, communicative ability with, or ultimate acceptance of a hearing aid's amplification. Accordingly, appropriate legislation is impossible to legislate these considerations.

A patient's ultimate acceptance of a hearing aid is more dependent upon their psychological adjustment to the amplification than upon any testing procedures. Accordingly, appropriate legislation concerning a patient's psychological adjustment to amplification is impossible.

A hearing aid is incapable of replacing any portion of the diseased auditory system. Its contribution is limited to its ability to amplify the input signals and to reproduce the frequencies of the input signals. Accordingly, a hearing aid cannot be expected to restore normal hearing, nor should its amplification be expected to be either pleasing or satisfying to a patient initially. On the basis of the limitations of the hearing aid, appropriate legislation is impossible.

When one places all of this data in proper perspective, the fact is that appropriate legislation concerning hearing aid evaluation and selection is not achievable at this time. Objective measurements must become accepted and methods of evaluating response must be accepted before legislation is possible.

Furthermore, one has to have serious reservations concerning the desirability of restrictive legislation in the hearing aid evaluation and selection process. In the majority of opinions, restrictive legislation at this time would only dampen research and development of new evaluation and selection systems which are desperately needed. Suppression of the infusion of new ideas would not be desirable at this time. Restrictive legislation would encourage restriction of new ideas.

The second abuse described is the concern for costs. Unfortunately, the cost issue was pressed by health care professionals, both physicians and clinical audiologists, who were poorly informed. They presented dispensing costs relative to their environments, which were primarily tax-supported, institution-supported, community-supported and physician-supported hearing centers. Such centers could not realistically approach the problems associated economically with hearing aid dispensing.

Unfortunately, the beneficial impact that could have influenced dispensing costs was lost because of the poorly advised statements. It would appear that the emphasis was upon the evaluation and selection rather than upon dispensing. In the field analysis, it became obvious that the cost relative to dispensing should minimize the evaluation process and emphasize more the support necessary to achieve a patient's psychological adjustment to amplification.

Of the three abuses, inappropriate fittings, unnecessary costs and the lack of medical attention, only the third, placing hearing aids upon persons who should have had medical treatment prior to the purchase of a hearing aid, could be consistently and objectively documented. Furthermore, the medical examination could be effectively legislated with uniform and consistent standards. The desirability of protecting an individual's best medical interests was obvious. Consequently, the desirability of the medical examination prior to the purchase of the hearing aid became law.

It is regrettable that the intent of the medical examination prior to the purchase of a hearing aid has been misrepresented. The intent of the medical examination is only to identify the medical parameters and establish medical diagnoses prior to the purchase of the hearing aid. The intent of the medical examination is not related to establishing a patient's candidacy for a hearing aid, other than on the basis of the presence or absence of medical disease which would contraindicate the application of a hearing aid.

The word "candidate" as used in legislation means only that an individual has been medically examined and may be considered for a hearing aid. One must always keep in mind that an individual cannot be forced to receive medical treatment. For example, merely because a patient has otosclerosis does not mean that she cannot receive a hearing aid. The otosclerosis could be treated medically or surgically, but the patient need not be forced to receive that treatment. The law merely states that the identification process must exist prior to the purchase of the hearing aid to protect the patient's best medical interests.

How should the physician respond to the responsibility of examining a patient medically prior to the purchase of a hearing aid? What should the physician performing the examination be capable of offering to the hearing handicapped individual?

First, an appropriate medical examination should be performed. There has been some justifiable criticism of the manner in which the medical examination is performed, relative to its thoroughness.

An appropriate medical examination implies obtaining a knowledgeable history, performing and interpreting an adequate physical examination of the ears, nose and throat and the assimilation of information obtained from hearing tests, which describe the type of hearing loss possessed by the patient.

The history will explore the differences in the hearing losses in the pre-language development period as well as in the post-language development period. In the pre-language development period, questions should inquire into genetic problems, such as Alexander, Michel, Mondini and Schiebe Aplasia of the inner ear, and genetic hearing losses associated with other system abnormalities, such as pupil color, hair color, skin pigmentation, thyroid disease, heart abnormalities, retinal pigmentation abnormalities, skeletal defects and renal problems.

Following the genetic history, inquiry into the mother's first twenty weeks of pregnancy is necessary. Viral infections, high fevers, rashes, ototoxic medications, radiation exposure and thyroid disease can all influence the development of the fetus during the first twenty weeks of life.

The next inquiry should be into the delivery. Was the delivery premature, or complicated by bleeding, jaundice, RH problems, anoxia, long labor or birth trauma.

Following this questioning, the possibility of mental retardation, autistic behavior, cerebral palsy or aphasia must be considered as well as cochlear disease.

The physical examination of the ears, nose and throat and appropriate studies must consider the examination of the ears, nose and throat as well as the other organ abnormalities that may be associated with genetic problems.

Concerning the reliability of hearing testing in pre-language development children, there is still considerable debate as to its effectiveness. Most authorities agree that a knowledgeable audiologist, in play or observation audiometry is preferable to the newer electronic evaluation systems, such as evoked auditory potentials, brain stem potentials or cochleography.

All of these studies have made significant contributions to the difficulties in establishing a diagnosis of hearing loss in the pre-language development child, but clinical acceptance is not reliable at this time.

How about questions relative to post-language development hearing loss? There are genetic causes for post-language development hearing losses, such as familial sensorineural hearing loss, otosclerosis, and hearing loss associated with other systemic abnormalities, such as skin pigmentation, eye pigmentation, skull abnormalities, renal abnormalities and central nervous system disorders.

Many infections influence hearing loss in the post-language development period, such as otitus media, labrynthitis, meningitis, encephalitis, viruses and syphilis. Non-infectious processes such as serous otitus media, ototoxicity, serious systemic illnesses, renal disease inner ear trauma by either noise exposure or direct head blows, thyroid disease and presbyacusis must be investigated. Other problems such as sudden hearing loss, Meniere's disease, inner ear fistulas, must be considered as well.

The hearing tests of pure tone air and bone conduction thresholds, speech and site-of-lesion testing, are helpful to the physician by describing the type of hearing loss possessed by the patient.

It becomes necessary that we stop for a moment and discuss the difference between discribing a patient's type of hearing loss and establishing the medical cause for the hearing loss. Hearing tests are capable of establishing a patient's type of loss but they're incapable of offering a medical diagnosis. It is for this reason that the medical examination by a physician, preferably one knowledgeable in the diseases of the ear, is essential prior to the purchase of a hearing aid. The performance of hearing tests, without a medical examination, is only capable of describing the individual's type of hearing loss, and not the medical cause for it.

For this reason, there is considerable discussion concerning the payment for pure tone threshold determinations, speech testing, and site-of-lesion testing prior to the purchase of the hearing aid. These hearing tests are meaningless without a medical examination. Therefore, they should not be performed in the absence of a medical examination. Secondly, these hearing tests contribute no information concerning a patient's amplification requirements unless the dispenser uses Dr. Berger's method of establishing amplification needs. Dr. Berger uses the pure tone air threshold determinations and applies a conversion formula to establish the individual's amplification needs on a frequency by frequency basis.

Accordingly, the use of pure tone threshold determination, speech testing and site-of-lesion testing are very important parts of the medical examination, but without the medical examination, are meaningless relative to establishing a patient's amplification requirements.

Following the medical examination and establishing the medical diagnosis, the physician should possess the knowledge necessary to recommend appropriate hearing aid evaluation and selection procedures. Many physicians may wish to perform this themselves, while others will prefer to send the patient to a Speech and Hearing Center for a hearing aid evaluation.

Rarely will the physicians themselves perform the tests, but their knowledge of the tests is essential for the physicians' intelligent guidance of the patient into the auditory rehabilitation process. As the hearing aid evaluation and selection procedure becomes more objective through quantitative measurements of a patient's psychoacoustic needs in amplification, the ability of the physician to more accurately participate in a knowledgeable manner in a patient's rehabilitation will increase. In addition to the physician's awareness of the need for more accurate hearing aid evaluation and selection procedures, there is an increasing awareness among the clinical audiologic profession that such improved hearing aid evaluation procedures are necessary. As a result, more accurate, reliable, and scientific hearing aid evaluation and selection procedures are evolving.

The physician will need the answers to four questions concerning a hearing aid's selection:
1. Has the best appropriate hearing aid been supplied?
2. Has the best dollar value been obtained in the dispensed hearing aid?
3. Does the individual possess reliable hearing aid consumer protection procedures by being able to compare one hearing aid with another in measureable terms?
4. When is a replacement hearing aid necessary?

Few disagree with the inadequacies inherent in hearing aid evaluation and selection procedures, relative to providing information required in the future. In addition, most otolaryngologists and clinical audiologists, as well as hearing aid dealers, knowledgeable with the problems of future hearing aid dispensing, are encouraging the development of hearing aid evaluation and selection procedures that measure the amplification requirements on a frequency by frequency basis. Such measureable expressions of amplification requirements enable more effective definition of roles, as well as security professionally within these roles. The physician will no longer feel the need to sell hearing aids in their offices. The physician can accurately establish the amplification requirements of the patient and provide them to a dispenser in a prescription form. In addition, once the hearing aid has been applied, the patient can return to the physician for more testing to make certain that the amplification goals of the hearing aid have been established. In such a way the physician can feel secure in knowing that the most effective amplification has been applied to his patient.

In this respect, the effectiveness of the clinical audiologist will be increased. They will be able to establish the amplification requirements of the patient in measureable terms, as well as participate in the actual sale of the hearing aid if they so wish. The acceptance of the clinical audiologist's participation in the hearing aid selection and sales process will be improved because the referring individual may know the accuracy of the hearing aid that has been dispensed. Furthermore, the dispensing agent, whether the manufacturer, hearing aid dealer, or clinical audiologist, will know that the aid they dispensed was the appropriate aid according to the recommendations of the individual who evaluated and selected the patient's amplification requirements.

Perhaps the most significant advantage of the selection of hearing aids on a frequency by frequency basis is the knowledge that those numerical standards will be valid in Chicago, Dallas, Paris, or Mexico City, regardless of dialect differences.

How can these frequency by frequency measurements fulfill the four goals established earlier relative to the needs of the evolving hearing aid dispensing programs?

First, the amplification requirements of the patient are established on a frequency by frequency basis, with numerical terms. The "prescription" is then provided to the manufacturer who can provide an appropriate hearing aid. Finally, when a patient wears the hearing aid, the patient can return for more testing to be sure that the desired amplification requirements have been fulfilled. In such a way, the physician, the clinical audiologist, hearing aid dispenser, and manufacturer are informed relative to the appropriateness of the fitting.

If the appropriate hearing aid has fulfilled the amplification needs, then the best dollar value has been obtained. Other sales measures may not be necessary.

When the patient has been evaluauted wearing the hearing aid, they can be given a graph of the performance of that hearing aid, which they can use to compare with other hearing aids' performances. If another aid can provide more frequencies, more effectively, then it would be a more appropriate hearing aid. By such measurements, the patient is offered an objective method of comparing one hearing aid's performance with another.

Finally, one of the critical needs of the evolving hearing aid dispensing programs is knowledge as to when another hearing aid is required. By such testing, one will be able to establish if a replacement hearing aid is necessary. If another hearing aid is capable of providing additional frequencies more effectively to the individual, then the individual is entitled appropriately to a replacement hearing aid.

The clinical audiologist must provide research and development environments to establish concepts such as Dr. Berger's method of converting pure tone threshold measurements into amplification requirements on a frequency by frequency basis, Dr. Victoreen's method of otometric measurements, Dr. McCandless' method of employing the acoustic reflex to establish amplification requirements on a frequency by frequency basis, Dr. Pascoe's method of establishing quantitatively, the hearing aid amplification requirements.

What is desirable in the hearing aid evaluation process is the development of a test signal that has a frequency by frequency capability of measuring some phenomenon in the normal ear which can be measured in a deficient ear and used to establish the amplification requirements in the deficient ear necessary to restore the deficient ear functionally to the normal ear, on a frequency by frequency basis. Speech testing simply cannot provide this information. Following the knowledge that the appropriate hearing aid has been selected, and that the patient has been evaluated wearing the hearing aid to determine that the appropriate and desired amplification goals have been achieved, the physician should be certain that the patient receives the hearing aid at a realistic cost and that appropriate service to support the instrument is provided by the vendor.

It is my sincere belief that physicians should not sell hearing aids. It is inappropriate and inconsistent with existing laws. In the FDA regulation concerning hearing aids, the patient is mandated to see a physician for a physical examination and medical evaluation of the hearing loss prior to the purchase of a hearing aid. When a patient is mandated by law to see a physician before the purchase of a hearing aid, it is inappropriate that the physician sell the hearing aid. There is no other prosthetic instrument which requires by law that the individual receiving the prosthetic instrument receive a medical examination prior to receiving the prosthetic instrument.

Accordingly, hearing aids should not be sold by physicians unless that physician declares himself as a hearing aid dealer and so sells hearing aids.

Fortunately, with the evolution of hearing aid evaluation and selection procedures which establish a patient's amplification requirements on a frequency by frequency basis, and which provide a mechanism of establishing whether appropriate or desirable amplification goals have been achieved following the application of the hearing aid, the physician can no longer state that it is necessary to sell the hearing aid from their offices in order to be certain that the patient is not either abused by inappropriate hearing aid application or abused by unreasonable charges for the hearing aid. The more objective frequency by frequency evaluation procedures will provide the physician and clinical audiologist the capability of "prescribing" the amplification requirements and establishing whether or not the appropriate amplification goals have been achieved.

Following the purchase of a hearing aid, the patient's physician should provide information concerning the appropriate personnel to assist that patient in psychologically adjusting to their hearing aid's amplification. The opportunity for a patient to ultimately accept amplification is poor, regardless of the severity of their hearing loss, if they do not recieve the appropriate counseling regarding their hearing aid's performance, its amplification capability and the relative limitations provided the individual by the amplification. Merely placing the hearing aid upon the individual that provides appropriate amplification does not exclude the responsibility of the dispensing agent from helping the individual adjust to the amplification. The patient must be encouraged relative to motivation, insight into their problem, and the limited measures available to assist their problems and provide their families, as well as the individual, with methods of auditory training in order to assist the individual to hear more effectively with their hearing aid.

The physician should be knowledgeable in the importance of insisting that their patients receive psychological support and be certain that the mechanism is provided in their community so that the patient may receive appropriate psychological aupport.

Finally, the physician who participates in the placement of hearing aids upon the hearing handicapped individuals should be knowledgeable relative to the additional communicative tools which might assist the patient to communicate more effectively with their hearing aid. The limitations provided by amplification are recognized by everyone, or at least should be, if those individuals are to participate in hearing aid dispensing programs.

Furthermore, the majority of people who will benefit from the evolving hearing aid dispensing programs will be the elderly, who spend many lonely hours without communicative abilities. By providing additional communicative aids to assist these people in their communication, one may provide more enjoyment instead of otherwise lonely hours. Specifically, these individuals enjoy watching television. There has been considerable discussion regarding the merits of sign language and its application to television. Can these elderly people be taught sign language effectively? Can the small size of the interpreter present on the screen provide adequate visual clues to the individual watching? Or would it be better to provide written captions? The physician should be actively participating in encouraging such communicative aids to assist the hearing handicapped in the community who wear a hearing aid.

I have been told by many individuals that the elderly reject amplification. This has not been my experience in a recent study. It is not that the elderly have rejected amplification, but that the elderly have been rejected. The elderly live in a world of silence and loneliness and receive no counseling. They fear the cost of hearing aids and the cost necessary to support the hearing aid. Few, if any, are ever offered any counseling which would help to bring them out of their world of silence. They have only been "sold" a hearing aid. This practice must stop.

The physician should be actively participating in assuring all hearing handicapped individuals receive the appropriate amplification, the psychological support necessary to assist them in accepting that amplification and in providing additional auditory aids which will assist them in utilizing more effectively their accepted amplification in their environment.

To achieve the physician's role in auditory rehabilitation, educational programs are necessary which do not exist presently. It would be my hope that the practicing otolaryngologist and the practicing audiologist would work cooperatively to achieve, as well as provide, appropriate auditory rehabilitation and training programs, not only for the patients, but for the professionals concerned with the rehabilitation of the patient. This specifically refers to physicians in communities. Regrettably, our academic centers provide our educational program and most academic centers have individuals who are removed from the realities of placing hearing aids upon patients. The academic professional can provide information concerning "how it should be done" but rarely provide answers to the problems of why an individual doesn't accept the hearing aid. Rarely can the academic person provide answers concerning patient acceptance of hearing aids.

It is with delight that I accept the news that an increasing number of clinical audiology training programs are actively participating in the dispensing of hearing aids. Previously, those individuals were concerned with the evaluation and recommendation of appropriate amplification, but never saw the end result of those appropriate recommendations. With the participation of the clinical audiologist in the actual dispensing programs, the reality of getting patients to accept hearing aids will become part of their professional activity. Education is the answer and through education, insecurities will be removed and the feeling of one professional being threatened by another will be eliminated.

Chapter 2

New Concepts in
Signal Processing and Hearing Rehabilitation

Paul Yanick, Jr., M.A.

Despite the vast amount of conflicting opinions as to what constitutes the optimum electro-acoustic characteristics for a given hearing impaired patient, Audiology is still struggling with a morass of unresolved problems, endless controversies, and inaccurate methods of arriving at the optimum in hearing aid fittings. As a clinical audiologist in private practice, I am convinced that many of these problems are directly related to our lack of close contact and feedback with the patient. Traditional approaches to providing compensatory amplification neglect the dynamics of the communicative events. Today's audiologist hardly ever see the dramatic effects that changing earmold acoustics, varying frequency-gain characteristics, and changing output limiting levels have on a hearing aid wearer in real-life situations. The vast amount of knowledge required to yield the optimum hearing for a client requires close feedback from the client himself. Knowing that because of a specific electro-acoustic manipulation or alteration, we have achieved some desirable or undesirable effect. The audiologist who inserts himself between the Otolaryngologist and hearing aid dealer fails to realize that the provision of effective counseling services and feedback with the patient are vital elements needed in maximizing total services to individuals with hearing impairments.
One of the main objectives of this chapter is to discuss some general critieria which may, at the present time, facilitate a reassessment of our current thinking regarding hearing aids and rehabilitation activities for sensorineural hearing loss. Practical suggestions and procedures are aimed

primarily at the clinical Audiologist who is confronted daily with the reality of providing appropriate rehabilitation services for patients with sensorineural hearing loss.

In investigating the possible effect of a given hearing aid on a hearing impaired individual a strong case as to the casual nature of an association between electro-acoustics and real world performances can often be built from observational evidence. In the absence of controlled experiment, however, it is possible always to doubt the casual nature of an association and to offer other explanations of the observations. When controlled experiment is not possible and we rely strongly on subjective data for our observation evidence, demand for absolute proof is highly unrealistic. A critical point of view in interpreting observational relationships as casual is prudent, but at some point in the accumulation of evidence it becomes wiser to accept the casual hypothesis as a basis for action than to continue to debate its validity. When controversy focuses on an unrealistic demand for absolute proof of one hypothesis or the other instead of limiting the discussion to where the point of controversy lies, our progress in solving many of the problems that face us regarding hearing aid applications is often limited and subdued. Observational evidence that results from years of feedback from all types and degrees of hearing loss, can result in clinical experience and knowledge that would allow Audiology to become a more proficient and viable profession.

Assessment of Communicative Function

Recently, several authors have investigated how people go about functioning in communicative situations in the auditory world (Kapteyn, 1977, 1977; Tonning, 1978). This approach demands that the patient receive adequate counseling, orientation and follow-up, an area that has been long neglected in the aural rehabilitation process. A report of considerable significance to the present endeavor is that of Tonning (1978). This author introduces the report by acknowledging that conventional speech audiometry does not provide realistic information concerning the desirable electro-acoustics of a given hearing aid in everyday listening conditions. He concludes that "we need to pay attention to the patient's experience with hearing aids under everyday listening conditions in each individual case when a hearing aid is selected".

Kapteyn (1977) and Kasten (1978) present views that success in adult aural rehabilitation with a hearing aid should be aimed at providing information not only to the individual but all family members as well. Counseling, orientation and follow-up visits should provide the hearing aid wearer and his family with necessary guidelines during adjustment and learning process of wearing a hearing aid.

As an audiologist in private practice, I have found that counseling hearing impaired patients is a necessary and vital element in maximizing the effectiveness of a particular hearing rehabilitation service. Audiologists are now beginning to recognize that counseling and routine follow-ups are essential services that certainly deserve extensive attention and further implementation. Recent chapters in audiology textbooks by Goetzinger, Sanders, Pollack, and Stream and Stream reflect the trend toward an increased delivery of counseling services by Clinical Audiologists.

Profile Rating Study

In a recent article, Yanick (1978) looked at the rehabilitative success rate of hearing aid use in real-life situations by using a profile rating questionnaire. The questionnaire was individually designed based on each patient's listening environments. The purpose of this study was to determine the extent to which current hearing aid fitting procedures were failing to meet the needs of each individual patient in real-life situations.

Eighty monaural hearing aid wearers subdivided into two groups of 40 each were evaluated with sound field techniques, unaided, with their conventional aid, and with an aid fit to obtain a uniform hearing level (UHL) response (Pascoe, 1975). Profile ratings were obtained for both their own and the UHL response aid over a 60 day period. Each subject evaluated the aid during this 60 day period and kept a record of listening difficulties as they occurred. In addition, all subjects answered the questionnaire on a weekly basis. After the 60 day period another aid was substituted and the same 60 day evaluation was repeated. Half the subjects evaluated their own aids first and the other half evaluated the UHL response aid first.

The results of the unaided and aided sound field measurements are shown in Figures 1a and 1b for both groups of subjects. If we compare their aided thresholds with the normal audibility curve we can clearly see that they are receiving too much low frequency energy. In other words, there is an imbalance between low and high frequency sensitivity thresholds. These imbalances failed to provide adequate compensation for the accentuated high frequency loss, and aggravated recruitment and tolerance problems considerably. This

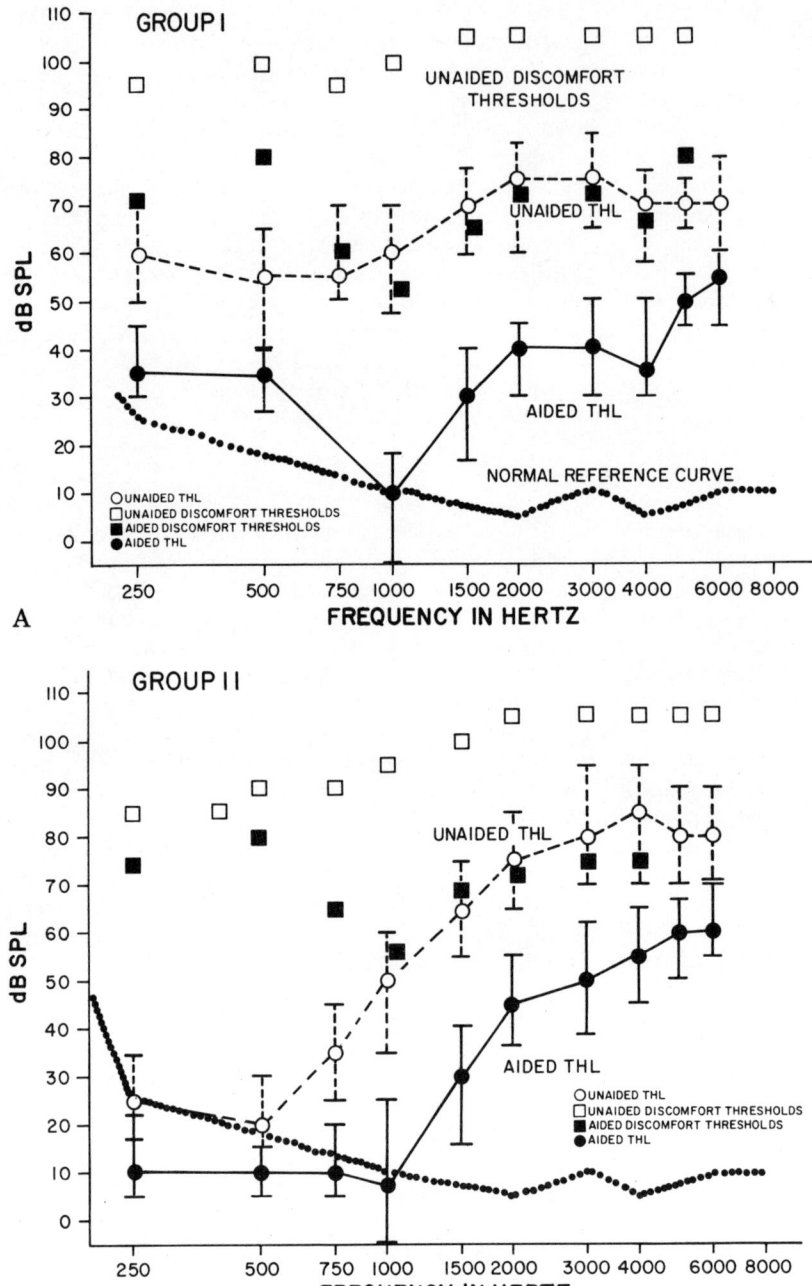

Figures 1a and 1b. Unaided and aided sound field measurements for both groups of subjects.

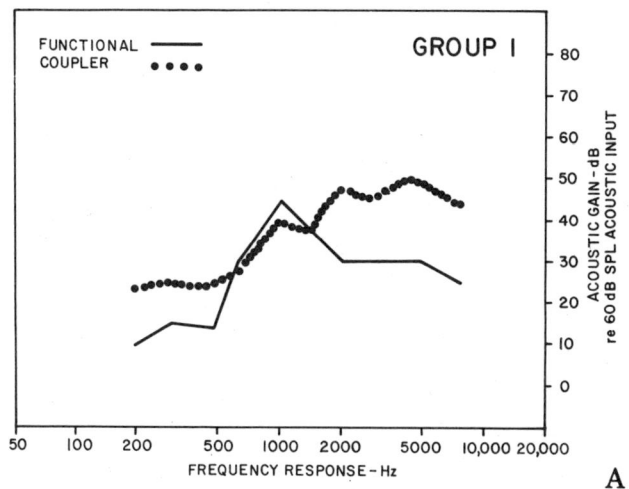

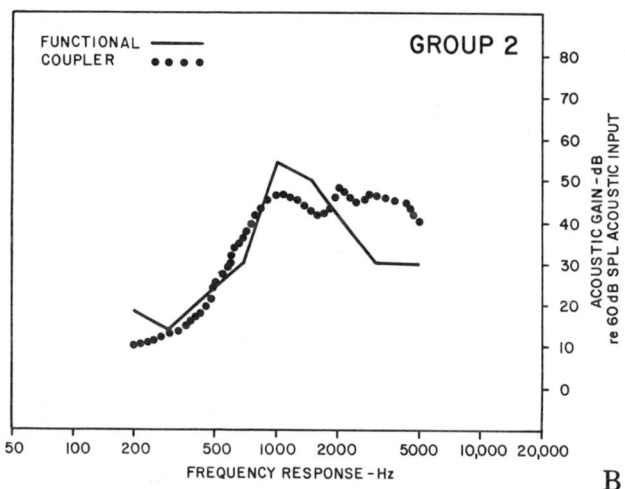

Figures 2a and 2b. Mean functional and coupler response for Groups I and II. (Reprinted by permission from Hearing Aid Journal, October 1978 issue.)

effect is clearly demonstrated by the aided discomfort thresholds shown in Figures 1a and 1b. The peaked functional gain in the vicinity of 1000 Hz caused aided discomfort thresholds to occur at input sound pressure levels of only 55 dB.

Figures 2a and 2b display the mean responses defined as functional and 2cc coupler gain for Groups I and II, respectively. Notice that the functional gain curves show a peaked region in the vicinity of 1000 Hz with poor high frequency

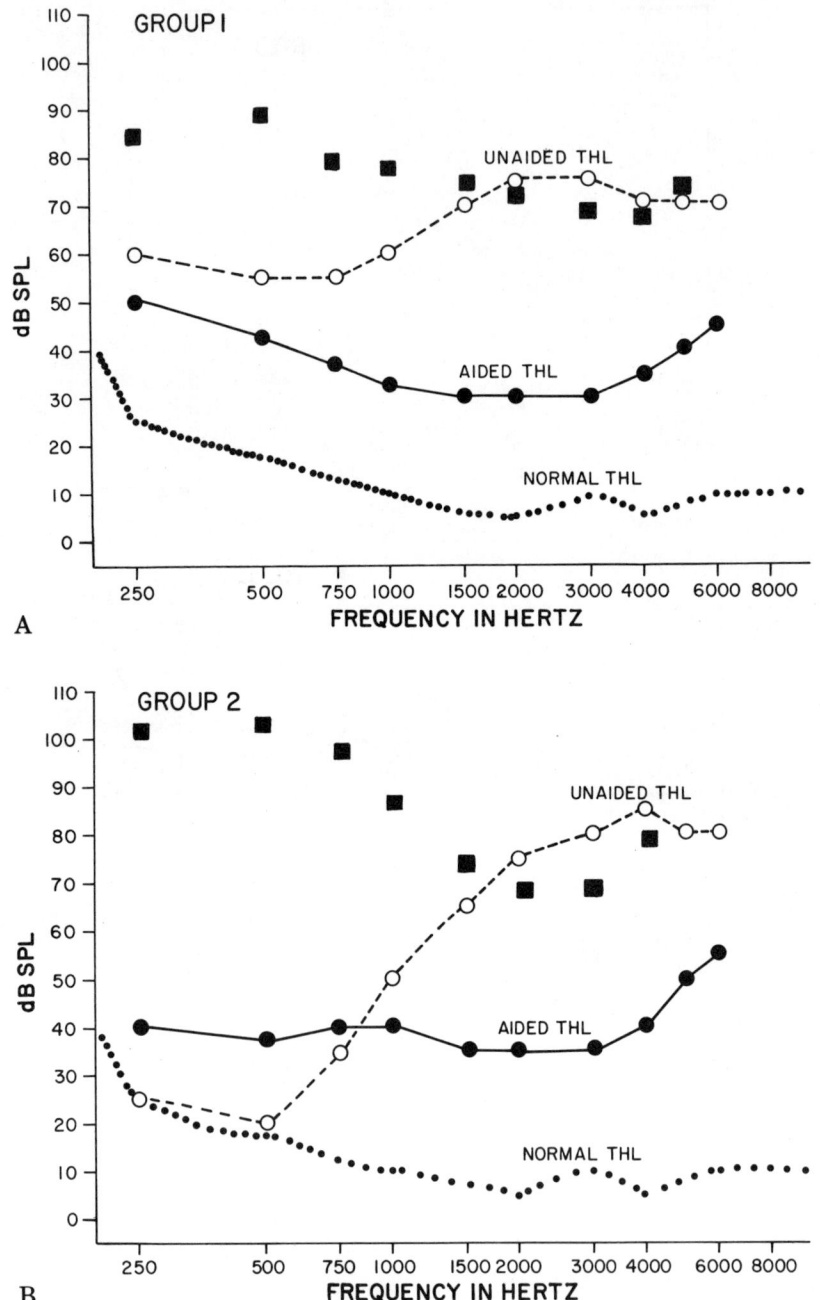

Figures 3a and 3b. Mean unaided and aided threshold measurements (Groups I and II) for the aid with a UHL response.

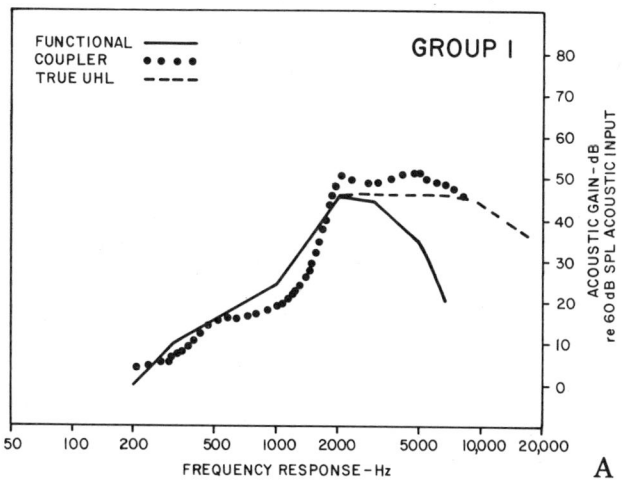

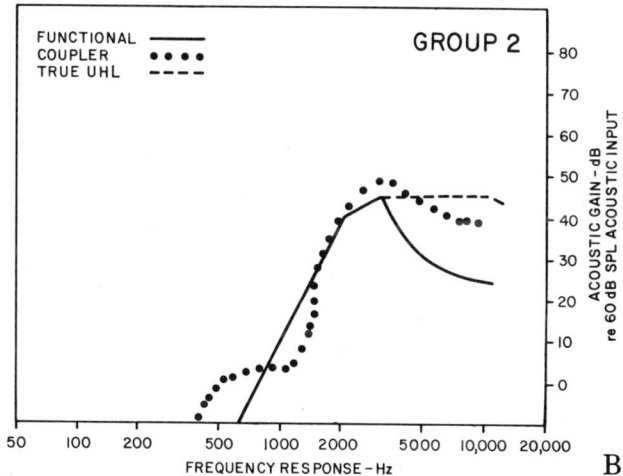

Figures 4a and 4b. Mean functional and coupler response for Groups I and II (shaped UHL response) and response needed to obtain an exact UHL response. (Reprinted by permission from Hearing Aid Journal, October 1978 issue.)

response. Conversely, the coupler measurements tend to overestimate functional gain in the 2 to 4 KHz region and underestimate functional gain in the .75 to 1.8 KHz region. These findings are in close agreement with Pascoe's (1975) findings for a group of subjects with similar hearing losses as those previously displayed in Group I (Figure 1a).

Figures 3a and 3b display the mean unaided threshold

measurements and the mean aided threshold measurements (Group I and II) for the aid with a UHL response. Notice that a true UHL response was not obtained. This was due to the performance limitations of the wearable aids used in this study and the relatively good unaided low frequency thresholds for subjects in Group II. The aided discomfort thresholds are also plotted for both groups in Figures 3a and 3b. Notice that they have shifted upward as much as 20 to 30 dB at frequencies centered around 1000 Hz.

Figures 4a and 4b reveal the mean functional gain and 2cc coupler gain responses for Groups I and II, respectively. The difference in decibels between functional and coupler gain responses was relatively constant for the subjects own aid (Figures 2a and 2b) and the aid with the UHL response. The true UHL response is also depicted in the figure to demonstrate the relatively poor high frequency response of today's hearing aids as compared with the desired response at frequencies above 2500 Hz.

The value of measuring functional gain for the purpose of obtaining a UHL response for each individual subject is clearly demonstrated by the dramatic differences in quiet and noisy real-life listening situations. The results are summarized in Tables 1 and 2.

Table 1.
The mean results of the profile rating for the quiet communicative situations for Group I and Group II.

	little or no difficulty understanding	some difficulty (but not a lot)	a fair amount of difficulty (quite a lot)	great difficulty in understanding
Group I				
own aid	5%	15%	40%	40%
new aid	55%	30%	15%	0%
Group II				
own aid	10%	20%	25%	45%
new aid	70%	20%	10%	0%

(Tables 1 and 2 reprinted by permission from Hearing Aid Journal, October 1978 issue.)

Table 2.
The mean results of the profile rating for the noisy communicative situations for Group I and Group II.

	little or no difficulty understanding	some difficulty (but not a lot)	a fair amount of difficulty (quite a lot)	great difficulty in understanding
Group I				
own aid	0%	10%	30%	60%
new aid	10%	60%	20%	10%
Group II				
own aid	0%	0%	45%	55%
new aid	5%	75%	15%	5%

Despite the improvements in hearing aids over the past 30 - 40 years it becomes evident that they have failed to provide adequate compensation for sensorineural hearing loss. Their failure in part is due to our inability to identify desirable electro-acoustics and the relatively inaccurate representation that 2cc coupler measurements have given us.

Coupler measurements (2cc) do not adequately reflect real-ear performance. This is evidenced by the work of several researchers (van Eysbergen and Green, 1959; Studebaker and Zachman, 1970; Tonnisson, 1975; McDonald and Studebaker, 1970; Pascoe, 1975; Yanick, 1978). The variability of individual ears necessitates real-ear performance measures which account for the acoustic effects of the ear mold, ear canal and pinna.

Even measurements made with the Kemar Manikin do not accurately reflect real-ear performance on a given individual. Kemar measurements can only simulate average real-ear performance. The point is clearly illustrated in Figure 5 on two different subjects yielding considerably different responses with the same hearing aid. Ear canal shape, length, and diameter, can unmistakeably change real-ear performance from individual to individual.

From the foregoing discussion, it is evident that real-ear performance measures must be collected in order to predict with some degree of confidence what the acoustic and amplification effects will have on the desired electro-acoustic output signal on a given individual. Adjusting the hearing aid so that it best meets the needs of each individual patient can give us a more valuable starting point for the fitting procedure. It can help us sort out known and documented un-

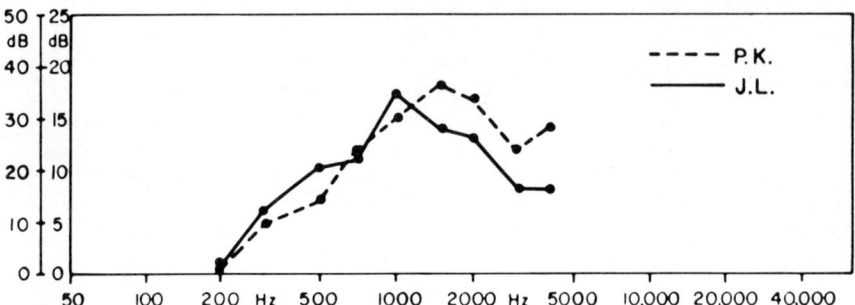

Figure 5. Results of tests on two different subjects using the same hearing aid.

desirable electro-acoustics and give us indications of how to proceed with our counseling activities.

Many current sound field techniques were developed at a time when precise electro-acoustic measurements of real-ear response were unknown. Some of these techniques have been discarded, others have been confirmed, and others await further study to determine the validity of the procedures employed. Desirable electro-acoustics is the goal we must set in each fitting procedure. Although optimum electro-acoustics is the ultimate goal it is still in the future and it awaits the results of many more scientific studies.

The decision to identify desirable electro-acoustics can be best facilitated by the use of controlled sound field measurements, variable and versatile wearable master hearing aids, a knowledge of earmold acoustics and an appropriate measure of the effectiveness of our efforts.

Sound Field Measurements

Sound field techniques can be used as a method of providing gain to compensate for the unaided hearing threshold levels. These measurements require careful consideration as they can unmistakeably lead to inaccurate results. The value and efficacy of our obtained measurements will be determined by the following: 1) the kind and locus of measurement of the stimulus; 2) the method of obtaining a response; 3) the particular procedure employed; 4) the method of blocking or masking the non-test ear; 5) the type and control of the signal; 6) the nature of the instructions given to the listener and 7) the rules we use to determine what it is we want in terms of a real-ear response.

The functional frequency-gain characteristics can be assessed by comparing the aided with unaided thresholds for each individual patient in sound field. Providing frequency selective amplification to provide compensation for unaided threshold levels does not mean that the aided threshold level must be placed directly on or close to the normal hearing threshold reference curve. This faulty assumption taken by a number of clinicians results in discomfort for supra-threshold stimuli, particularly when recruitment and a narrow dynamic range of hearing is present. Thus, the frequency-gain characteristics of a hearing aid should follow closely the contour of the normal reference curve, but the overall gain must be less than the overall hearing loss (Yanick, 1978; Pascoe, 1975). Threshold of discomfort measurements can assist us in determining how much less the overall gain will be. While this method works well for mild to moderately severe flat to gradual sloping sensorineural hearing losses, it must be modified somewhat when dealing with sharp sloping severe high frequency hearing loss (Skinner, 1976).

According to Skinner (1976), the best frequency response for subjects having a noise-induced severe high frequency loss was found to be that in which there was a 0 dB gain below 500 Hz and 23 dB at 1.6 KHz and above. The slope of the functional gain between 500 Hz and 1.6 KHz was followed by the difference between each subject's hearing threshold curve and the normal hearing threshold curve. There is also recent evidence (Yanick, 1978) that indicates high frequency gain in cases of severe high frequency losses will only add to existing perceptual distortions and decrease the intelligibility of speech. This topic will be covered in considerable detail later in this chapter.

Variable Response Electro-Acoustic Hearing Aids

In order to obtain the desirable functional gain response for each individual, we need to choose wearable hearing aids that are variable enough to permit the necessary adjustments. Variable frequency response and adjustable output levels are the most common forms of adjustments found on some of today's hearing aids. The more variable and versatile the aid, the closer we can get to a desired response.

Undesirable Electro-Acoustic Characteristics

As previously mentioned, there are known and documented undesirable electro-acoustic characteristics that we can look for when choosing a hearing aid. Dips and peaks in frequency response curves are known to decrease the listener's comfortable listening range, aggravate tolerance and recruitment problems by introducing formants which are a property of the hearing aid's response curve instead of the speech itself.

Intermodulation distortion (IMD) in hearing aids results with the interaction of two or more frequencies in a complex signal, such as speech. Both harmonic and IMD distortion arise from the same source, non-linearities. However, since harmonic distortion arises from a single tone, IMD measurements are of considerable importance because they represent a more realistic simulation of speech. Yet, very little is known about the contribution of IMD distortion to listeners performance with hearing aids.

The lack of correlation between amplifier distortion and listening tests have been noted by many audio-design engineers and researchers (Horowitz, 1964; Ashley, 1976; Leinowen, Otala and Curl, 1977; Schweitzer, Causey, and Tolten, 1977; Tremaine, 1973). Some conventional aids often measure under 10% Total Harmonic Distortion, yet they sound totally unacceptable, even though they are matched in terms of electro-acoustic characteristics. It appears therefore that audible differences between hearing aids may very well be contributed to forms of static and dynamic IMD levels. One author has suggested that approximately 3:1 IMD harmonic distortion can be expected in an audio amplifier. However, this ratio may be lower or higher depending upon the electro-acoustic characteristics of a particular hearing aid. Hence, it is difficult to use any formula based on HD levels. The aim of future research should be to quantitatively measure both static and dynamic forms of IMD and carefully observe their effect on speech processing through hearing aids.

Evidence strongly suggests that a decrease of the low frequencies at the tympanic membrane yields substantial improvements in speech intelligibility scores. Our daily contact with the hearing impaired person who constantly complains of noise as being highly disruptive to the communicative process should certainly support this evidence. Since most background noise is composed largely of low frequencies, decreasing low frequencies below 1500 Hz is certainly a desirable effect to achieve. Furthermore, it is well known that the most important frequency span for speech lies between 1500 and 2500 Hz.

By reducing low frequency levels and providing a smooth rising response, we also reduce IMD and HD levels considerably. If the primary peak of the hearing aid's response is at 2000 Hz instead of 750 Hz, multiples of 2000 Hz will very rapidly approach the high frequency cut-off point of the hearing aid which is an area of complete inaudibility. It is well known that amplified low frequencies rise much faster than amplified high frequencies causing a discomfort problem and high distortion levels to occur at saturation sound pressure levels.

Excessive low frequency amplification has been known to summate and interact unfavorably with distortions that occur in cochlear damaged ears. Yet, hearing aids continue to be manufactured with sharp peaked regions in frequency areas below 1500 Hz, and clinicians continue to fit them.

The input to the damaged cochlea (processed through a hearing aid) must be controlled, quantified, assesses and re-assessed more carefully than we have done in the past. The abnormal spread of masking from higher level low frequency components and the increased effective and critical bandwidth are known to result in deterioration in the ability of the damaged ear to detect signals in the presence of background noise.

Earmold Acoustics

Although there are relatively few aids available on the market that would enable us to obtain an exact UHL response, their application is often limited because of the vast array of hearing losses generated in the clinical population. Earmold acoustics can help us to improve the smoothness of a particular frequency response and extend the upper high frequency cut-off point. Killion (1978) discusses the effective methods of using acoustic damping elements to allow better smoothing of low frequency tubing resonances with improved high frequency output. He further suggests the addition of a stepped-bore in the earmold "horn coupler" to increase high frequency output in the 3 to 6 KHz region approximately 6 dB.

Recruitment Compensation

There are cases of sensorineural hearing loss that would

benefit from compression in addition to the above mentioned processing. When the dynamic range is narrow, amplified speech levels cannot fit properly between the threshold of hearing and discomfort levels. The result is that the listener receives an insufficient amount of acoustic speech cues that is often further degraded and masked by noise and acoustical interference.

Several authors (Villchur, 1973; Yanick, 1975; Barford, 1976) have suggested the use of multichannel compression combined with frequency equalization to compensate for recruitment. Although this system has tremendous potential for moderately severe hearing impairments, linear amplification combined with variable filtering and output limiting capabilities has proven to be reasonably successful for mild to moderate cases of sensorineural hearing loss.

Adaptive Filtering

Other processing routines have been proposed that vary the filtering characteristics of a hearing aid according to the overall input level (Yanick and Drucker, 1978). Listeners with sensorineural hearing loss have patterns of equal loudness contours in which specific frequency regions are attenuated depending upon the listening level. In other words, a UHL response may be adequate in the vicinity of sensitivity threshold, but may not adequately compensate for supra-threshold loudness function and discomfort thresholds. The most important factor that should be considered is the relative change in frequency response that occurs when the hearing aid user adjusts his volume control to provide for a comfortable listening level. If volume control rotation effectuated a frequency response change that would compensate for the accentuated frequency regions at different listening levels the hearing aid would process speech to yield optimum speech intelligibility scores at supra-threshold listening levels. The results of this study on twelve subjects revealed a significant increase in speech intelligibility scores at both a 65 and 85 dB SPL presentation level. In addition, this form of speech processing resulted in an increase of 6 dB gain at a 65 dB presentation level and 14 dB at an 85 dB presentation level.

Another more recent study (Long, 1979) has demonstrated that changing the functional gain response of a hearing aid at moderate and loud conversational speech can yield dramatic differences in the speech intelligibility scores of 10 listeners with sensorineural hearing loss. This study utilized aided and unaided threshold of discomfort levels to determine a functional-gain response at supra-threshold listening levels, and a UHL response at levels in the vicinity of sensitivity threshold.

Output Limitation

Another innovative approach to signal processing is Single Side Band (SSB) instantaneous amplitude clipping as a means of output limiting (Gregory and Drysdale, 1976). This method has been combined with multi-channel compression and also used with linear amplification (Yanick, Patent #890069). Splitting the speech signal into several frequency bands, and individually amplitude compressing each band according to the recruitment characteristics of each specific cochlear loss must be supplemented with some form of frequency equalization and output limiting. Ideally, output limiting would consist of SSB clipping that avoids distortion products by clipping them outside the speech band. This task is accomplished by modulating a high frequency carrier with the speech and then clipping the modulated carrier. The clipped components are now produced outside the transposed speech band and prevented from re-entering the speech band on de-modulation by filtering. Since the clipped amplitude peaks contribute little information as compared with the time intervals at the "cross-over" (zero) region, very little important speech information is lost. The most impressive performance of this signal processing scheme is that it avoids the problems of integration time contents and HD. However, recent research has shown that SSB should be combined with amplitude compression because when the "cross-over" (zero) region is superimposed on the peak excursions of higher uncompressed level signals many speech cues are lost by clipping.

Extended High Frequency Amplification

Recent research suggests that persons with sensorineural hearing impairment should derive extra benefit from extended high frequency amplification between 4000 and 6500 Hz (Long, 1979; Harrison, 1974). Such amplification seems to provide the impaired ear with additional speech cues, which is especially beneficial for optimal capability of utilizing these additional cues without added perceptual distortions.
I have found it inconcievable and unjustifiable to put aids on some subjects with spectral information beyond 4000 Hz, or for some cases even beyond 2000 Hz without carefully

assessing the potential of the cochlear damaged ear for receiving speech information in this spectral area. Extended high frequency amplification can produce compounding effects if the dynamic range is relatively narrow (difference between hearing loss and threshold of discomfort < 15dB).

I do not wish to imply that extended high frequency amplification is of no value to cochlear losses. I have evidence that an extended high frequency cut-off point can provide additional valuable information to some forms of cochlear losses. Conversely, if the cut-off slope extends beyond the point that high distortion levels occur in a specific spectral region we can expect a dramatic reduction in speech intelligibility to occur.

The following cases are presented to illustrate the importance of a variable high frequency cut-off frequency for some cases of cochlear losses:

Case 1 (Figure 6) is of a 29 year old female with a sharp sloping severe high-tone sensorineural hearing loss in the left ear, and a severe sensorineural hearing loss in the right ear. Her unaided discrimination score (DS) at a most comfortable listening level was measured at 34% in the left ear. This patient had been wearing a high frequency emphasis hearing aid on her left ear very unsuccessfully. She complained of hearing a constant hissing noise and unclear speech. Her aided DS was 22%, much poorer than her unaided score of 34%. A complete electro-acoustic evaluation of her hearing aid by conventional coupler methods could not substantiate her complaints of noise and unclear speech. Distortion levels were minimal and the internal noise levels of her aid were relatively low. After considerable experimentation, I cut-off the high frequencies above 2000 Hz and she noted that the hissing noise disappeared and the speech was much clearer. Her aided DS with a 2000 Hz cut-off was measured at 52%.

Case 2 (Figure 7) is of a 54 year old male who had similar complaints about his hearing aid. He had a bilateral accentuated high frequency hearing loss with an unaided DS of 54%, but he still claimed that he could hear better without his hearing aid. After modifying his aid's response to cut-off frequencies above 2500 Hz, his DS improved to 72% and he noticed an immediate improvement in his aided hearing ability.

A master hearing aid that can vary the high frequency cut-off point at ½ octave intervals between 2000 and 6500 Hz can provide invaluable information when assessing the potential of the impaired ear for utilizing speech information in this spectral area. Knowledge of each patient's dynamic range at these frequencies would necessitate that speech intelligibility tests be performed to determine an optimum high

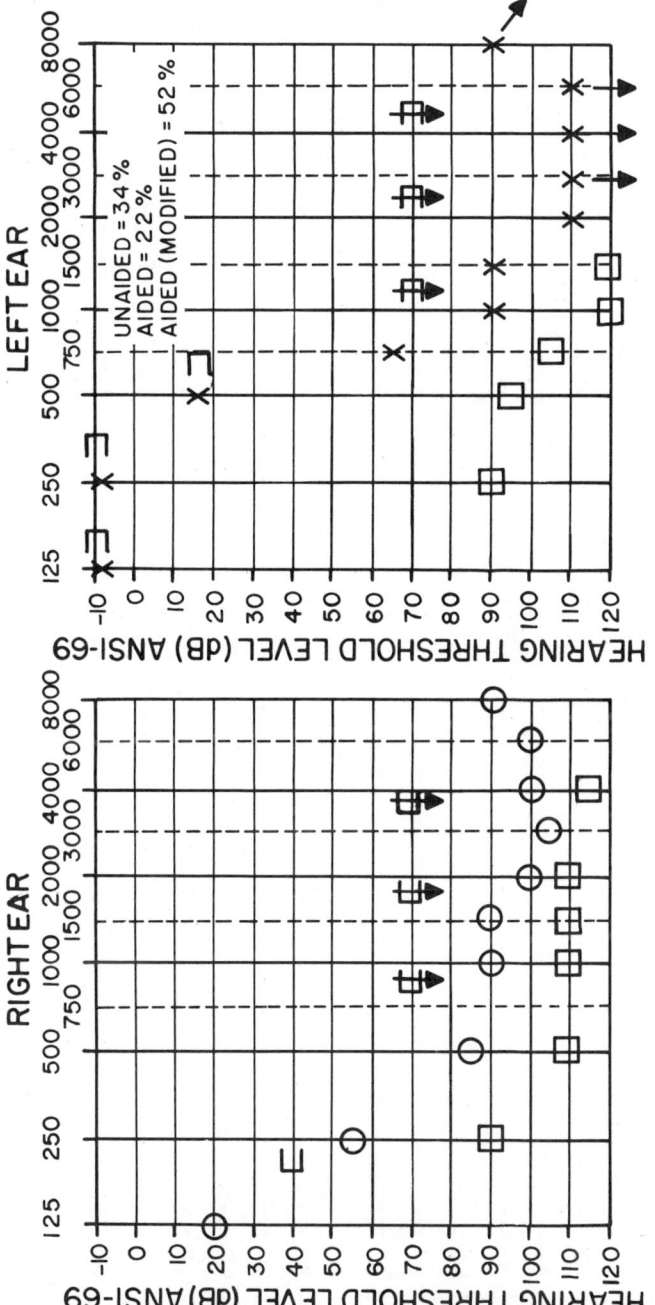

Figure 6. Case 1: a 29 year old female with bilateral sensorineural hearing loss. The squares indicate the discomfort thresholds.

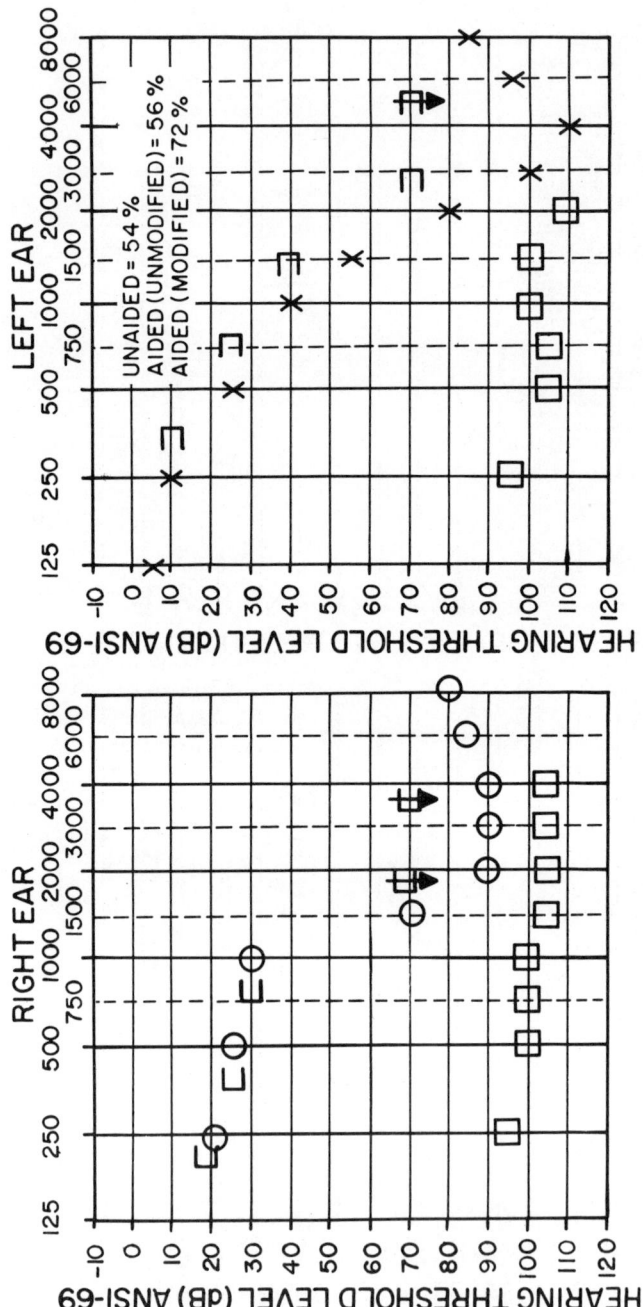

Figure 7. Case 2: a 54 year old male with bilateral sensorineural hearing loss. The squares indicate this subject's discomfort thresholds.

frequency cut-off point.

Conclusion

This chapter illustrates the importance of a total hearing rehabilitation process involving more than conventional audiological test procedures. We must become more aware of the desirable electro-acoustic characteristics of a hearing aid as they relate to a given hearing impaired person. Effective counseling and close patient feedback are vital ingredients that help us come closer to a more successful hearing aid fitting. Effective remediation warrants focusing on the communication process in a variety of real-life listening situations.

References

Ashley, R., On the audibility of distortion in loud speakers, Paper presented at IEEE International Conference on Acoustics, Speech, and Signal Processing, Phila., (1976).

Barford, J., Multi-channel compression hearing aids, The Acoustics Lab Tech. Report, No. 11, (1976).

Gregory, R.L. and Drysdale, A.D., Squeezing speech into the deaf ear, Nature, Vol. 264, No. 5588 748-751 (1976).

Harford, E.R. and Fox, J., The use of high-pass amplification for broad frequency sensorineural hearing losses, Audiology, 17, 10-26 (1978).

Harrison, A., The use of high frequency response hearing aids with moderate to severe hearing losses, Audecibel, 23, 137-144 (1974).

Horowitz, M., Intermodulation distortion - pros, cons, and hows, Audiology, 48, 38-42 (1964).

Kapteyn, T.S., Factors in the appreciation of a prosthetic rehabilitation, Audiology, 16, 446-452 (1977).

Kapteyn, T.S., Satisfaction with fitted hearing aids, Scand. Audiology, 6, 171-177 (1977).

Kasten, R.N. The hearing aid as related to rehabilitation, in the Handbook of Adult Rehabilitative Audiology, Ed. Alpiner, J.G., Williams and Wilkens, 67-87 (1978).

Killion, M.C., Problems in the application of wideband hearing aid earphones, Presented at Conference on Acoustic Factors Affecting Hearing Aid Measurement and Performance, City University of New York, (1978).

Leinowen, E., Otala, M. and Curl, J., A method for measuring transient intermodulation distortion, J. Aud. Eng. Soc., 25, 4, 170-177 (1977).

Long, L., Adaptive vs. fixed functional-gain response, submitted to Audiology and Hearing Education Journal for publication, (1979).

McDonald, F.D. and Studebaker, G.A., Earmold alteration effects as measured in the human auditory meatus, J. Acous. Soc. Amer., 48, 1366-1372 (1970.

Pascoe, D.P., Frequency response of hearing aids and their effect on the speech perception of hearing impaired subjects, Ann. Otol. Rhino. Lar., 84, Suppl. 23, No.5, 2 (1975).

Schweitzer, H.C., Causey, G.D. and Tolten, M.C., Nonlinear distortion in hearing aids: the need for re-evaluation of measurement philosophy and technique, J. Amer. Audiology Soc., Vol. 2:4, 132-141 (1977).

Skinner, M.W., Speech intelligibility in noise induced hearing loss: effects of high frequency compensation, Doctoral Dissertation, Washington University, (1976).

Studebaker, G.A. and Zachman, T.A., Investigation of the acoustics of earmold vents, J. Acoust. Soc. Amer., 4, 1107-1115 (1970).

Tonning, F.M., Evaluation of hearing aid fitting based on the patient's experiences from everyday listening conditions, Scand. Audiology, 7, 13-17 (1978).

Tonnisson, W., Measuring in-the-ear gain of hearing aids by acoustic reflex method, J. Speech Hear. Res., 18, 17-30 (1975).

Tremaine, H.M., Audio Cyclopedia, Howard Sams Co., Inc., Bobs-Merrill, New York, (1973).

van Eysbergen, H.C. and Groen, J.J., The 2 mi. coupler and the high frequency performance of hearing aids, Acoustica, 9, 381-386 (1959).

Villchur, E., Signal processing to improve speech intelligibility in perceptive deafness, J. Acoust. Soc. Amer., 53, 1646-1657 (1973).

Yanick, P., Effects of signal processing on intelligibility of speech in noise for persons with sensorineural hearing loss, J. Amer. Aud. Soc., 1:5, 229-238 (1975).

Yanick, P., The communicative function of hearing aid wearers in real-life situations, Hearing Aid Jour., Oct., (1978).

Yanick, P., Hearing aids using single-side banded clipping, Patent No. 890069.

Chapter 3

Electrostimulation of the Cochlea: A Brief History

James Martin, Ph.D.

Introduction

The first purpose of this report is to review the research relevant to the efficacy of the so-called (TD) transdermal therapy for sensorineural hearing loss. I will begin by reporting those studies which purport to shed light on the issue of efficacy. Secondly, I will evaluate the sometimes inconsistent finding of those as well as subsequent studies with an eye toward both resolving the apparent contradictions in the literature as well as characterizing the emerging pattern of results which is supported by this literature as a whole. In this context I will comment on a previous attempt to review this literature.

Third, I will summarize those findings which shed light on the conditions under which the TD therapy is likely to be effective. Fourth, I will describe data which suggest the character of the physiological basis for the efficacy of the transdermal therapy. I will describe the rationale which has been developed to explain the therapeutic effect of transdermal electrostimulation.

For well over a century it has been known that electrical currents, when placed across the head, can sometimes produce the sensation of sound. This phenomenon (called the <u>electrophonic effect</u>) was first noticed by both Volta and Fechner prior to the present century. More recently, it has been discovered that an amplitude modulated electromagnetic signal, when placed on the head, will produce the sensation of a sound with the same (or double) frequency of the amplitude modulation. Kelloway (1941, 1942) has demonstrated that this phenomenon is the result of an effect by virtue of which the tissues of the head are caused to vibrate by the alternating potential of the electrical current.

The discovery that electrostimulation has a therapeutic effect in persons with sensorineural hearing loss was made and reported by Puharich and Lawrence (1969). In exploring the possibility that the electrophonic effect could be used as the mechanism for a kind of hearing aid, Puharich and Lawrence discovered, quite accidentally, that persons with sensorineural loss, who were given daily exposures to electrostimulation, reported significant improvement in their ability to hear in everyday settings.

Puharich and Lawrence (1969) then executed and reported a double-blind study in which they found that TD therapy produced small improvements in some puretone thresholds and larger improvements in speech discrimination scores for subjects with sensorineural hearing loss. Their study was well controlled by normal scientific standards. It might have been immediately accepted had there been sufficient rationale for expecting the sorts of results they reported.

The unexpected character of their results led to extensive attempts to replicate. Five different groups of investigators executed double-blind experiments roughly approximating the procedures of Puharich and Lawrence. Three reported positive results, while two reported finding no effect. In retrospect, it is now apparent that methodological differences among the studies can be invoked to explain their different outcomes. One of the negative studies (Glattke and Simmons, 1974) is characterized by a number of procedural and conceptual errors. I think it can be shown beyond any doubt that the Glattke and Simmons' study is without scientific merit. The second negative result (Gerkin, Glorig & Roeser, 1974) was adequately designed. However, unknown to the investigators, the current they were administering to their subjects was being cut 62% by a switch box introduced to handle the peculiarities of the double-blind procedure. Thus, the initial negative results are now largely comprehensible in terms of an adequate understanding of experimental and statistical methodology and an increased understanding of the equipment used in those experiments.

Experimenters who obtained positive results appear to have been more concerned with therapeutic technique and delivered more therapeutic current to their subjects than those who failed to obtain results. Contrary to the opinion of Tonndorf (1974), a <u>careful</u> review of all these studies and the controversy which surrounded them shows that the TD therapy can be effective if reasonable methodological precautions are taken and if the subjects are given adequate therapy.

Considerable subsequent work on TD therapy has been carried out by Martin and his colleagues at Penn State University and Hughes and his colleagues at U.S.C. The result of this work has been to provide information concerning the parameter values necessary in order to observe optimal improvement. Also this information gives the basis for a rationale or explanation for the efficacy of the therapy.

In particular, one of the most important findings has been that the observed improvement is greatest in testing conditions in which there is competition between the to-be-perceived stimulus and noise (situations under which persons suffering with sensorineural loss report the greatest difficulty).

Further arguments and evidence are developed to support the view that TD therapy improves perception of speech by narrowing critical bands which have been pathologically widened.

This theory implicates the outer hair cells and their associated neural structures. These structures are thought to be responsible for narrowing the critical band. On the hypothesisthat pathology in these cells, causing them to be non-functional, is responsible for a widened critical band, it is suggested that TD therapy narrows critical bands by facilitating the metabolism of those cells. Two suggestions as to how TD therapy might improve cellular metabolism are supported by empirical work on the TD therapy.

Finally, I discuss work by Bochenek and Bochenek (1976) which demonstrates that TD therapy increases the amplitude of the auditory nerve action potential-- given the same amplitude auditory signal before and after therapy. It is universally recognized that this action potential is correlated in important ways with the possibility of hearing. The findings of Bochenek and Bochenek established a link between the TD therapy and physiological changes which may be plausibly related to improved hearing.

In summary, there were two sources of doubt which initially confronted the TD terapy-- a lack of rationale, and the inability of two early investigators to replicate Puharich and Lawrence's original findings. In this paper, I have given a rationale for the TD therapy which is grounded in a broad range of psychological and physiological literature. I have also shown that those initial failures to replicate the original findings probably resulted from a contribution of methodological deficiencies and imperfections in the equipment used in those early double-blind experiments.

Review and Evaluation of Research on Transdermal Therapy

There are three categories of work which have been variously reported and which shed light on transdermal therapy.

First, there were those studies which were aimed at rather directly assessing the efficacy of TD therapy in producing improvement of hearing in cases of sensorineural loss. In these studies, there was always some attempt to compare the performances of sensorineural patients after therapy with their own performance before therapy, on a variety of standard audiological perceptual tasks. Usually, there was an accompanying control group (double-blind), thus making possible a determination of the amount of change produced by the therapy and that which might result from either a placebo effect or experimenter bias. Typically, these evaluations were the first studies to be performed by each group of investigators. Sometimes, they were the only studies to be executed by a given group. Accordingly, with the exception of the original study by Puharich and Lawrence (1969), they were invariably carried out by investigators who were, at that time, essentially unfamiliar with the TD therapy. As will appear below, this fact may particularly account for the somewhat ambiguous results of these studies.

The second category of studies involves attempts to further understand the TD therapy. These studies, executed mostly by Hughes and his colleagues at the University of Southern California or by Martin and his colleagues at The Pennsylvania State University, generally presuppose the efficacy of the TD therapy. They represent attempts to develop our understanding of the TD therapy through variation of treatment parameters and the exploration of the effect as measured in terms of a number of different hearing tests.

The third group of studies to be reviewed here relate to the effect of TD therapy on the physiological mechanisms presumed to be related to hearing. These studies support a plausible link between TD therapy and improved hearing. First, it is argued that cochlear or retro-cochlear cells of persons suffering with sensorineural loss are not necessarily dead but may only be nonfunctional. Second, the general physiological effects of the therapy, increased blood flow and altered cell membrane potential, could benefit such nonfunctional cells. Third, it is shown that TD therapy increases the amplitude of the VIII nerve action potential. The full significance of this change is not yet known, but there is every reason to think that it should result in improved auditory functioning.

In this section I present a summary and analysis of studies intended to directly assess the efficacy of TD therapy.

As already stated, the initial demonstration of TD therapy was given by Puharich and Lawrence (1969). In that paper, Puharich and Lawrence reported the results of a double-blind investigation of the efficacy of the TD therapy. The degree of control for possible placebo or experimenter bias, which Puharich and Lawrence built into the design of their study, was exemplary. Neither the subjects, nor the therapists, nor the clinicians who evaluated the subjects' hearing both before and after therapy could have known which subjects were receiving therapy. Puharich and Lawrence reported finding no consistent evidence that TD therapy facilitated pure tone thresholds. However, they did find that TD therapy appeared to improve the perception of speech.

In view of the careful constraints they imposed on their experimental design, it is clear that the initial controversy surrounding their report stemmed from the wholly unexpected nature of their findings rather than from any carelessness in their experiment. It was no doubt felt that, in the absence of any plausible explanation for it at the physiological level, the effect must be shown to be extremely robust in order to be taken seriously. In what follows, it will be shown that we now know the conditions under which the TD therapeutic effect can be made to be reasonably robust and, moreover, that we can begin to locate some of the physiological systems in terms of which a full explanation for the effect is eventually likely to be framed. In fact, I will present a rationale for the efficacy of the therapy which is supported by both psychological and physiological data.

In order to develop this position, I will devote the majority of this section to discussing the five publicly reported attempts to replicate the Puharich and Lawrence findings.

Before beginning our account of these studies, however, it is necessary to describe the standard audiological tests and general procedures used in all of the investigations reported in this section. First, the pure tone threshold at a number of frequencies (characteristically 250, 500, 1000, 2000, 4000, and 8000 Hz) was usually taken for each ear. Second, and more important, each subject was tested (in each ear) for his ability to perceive speech. Typically, this was done by first determining the speech reception threshold (SRT) and subsequently the speech discrimination function. Characteristically, the speech discrimination function was determined in relation to amplitudes corresponding to SRT + 20dB, SRT + 30dB, and SRT + 40dB. Subjects either wrote or verbally repeated each word as it was presented.

It is important to note, in this connection, that while scores for presentation levels of SRT + 0dB through SRT + 30dB are more significant therapeutically than are changes at higher levels of amplitude.

The general procedure was as follows: with the exception of one study (Glattke and Simmons, 1974), subjects received 30 sessions of treatment. The treatment sessions lasted 50 minutes and were conducted 5 days per week. All subjects completed the treatment sessions in 7 weeks or less. After treatment, all subjects were reevaluated audiologically.

Each subject was seated at a table on which there was a TD-100 electrostimulation unit (manufactured by Intellectron Corporation). A technician placed a set of four electrodes on the subject's head, and dialed a number on a switch box which determined whether the experimental or the control condition was being presented. Each subject was assigned a number at the beginning of the experiment, and the number was always dialed for each subject at the beginning of each treatment session. Neither the subjects nor the technician knew the significance of the particular numbers. The subjects were simply told that the numbers represented different levels and modes of treatment. Because electrostimulation produces the sensation of sound, hidden earphones in the headsets produced subjectively identical sounds in the ears of placebo subjects. Thus, the procedures for experimental and placebo subjects were identical in every respect.

In this context, I begin with a discussion of the work of Hughes, Arthur, and Whitaker (1974). These authors report a preliminary evaluation of TD therapy involving three studies--one pilot study with 16 subjects and two double-blind studies with 28 and 19 subjects.

In the pilot study, the percentage of words repeated correctly increased (as a function of therapy) more in the lower ranges (above SRT) than at SRT + 40dB. The average gain at SRT + 30dB was 11%. At SRT + 20dB it was 16%, and at SRT + 10dB it was 25%. These changes are considerably greater than could be accounted for by the normal variability of hearing of sensorineural patients. Nevertheless, in the absence of a double-blind control group, it was impossible to be sure that the effect was not due to either placebo effects or experimenter biases.

Therefore, Hughes and his colleagues executed two double-blind experiments. (Because the audiologist was able to guess which subjects were in the experimental group on the basis of the subjects' spontaneous introspective reports of improvement Hughes et al. (1974) erroneously refer to one of these studies as single-blind. However, since neither the experimenter nor the subjects in either experiment had any information, other than the actual improvement on the subject, that would discriminate between active and placebo conditions, it is quite proper to call both of these experiments double-blind.) The results of these two experiments supported the hypothesis that the TD therapy is effective in improving hearing in some cases of sensorineural loss. In the first double-blind experiment there's an average improvement in the experimental group of 11% in speech discrimination scores at all intensities of presentation except SRT + 40dB. The placebo group improved 1% for the same intensities. The evidence showed a strong experimental effect and a negligible placebo effect. The difference was significant ($p < .02$).

In the second double-blind experiment, evaluating at intensity level SRT + 10dB, the active group improved 19% and the placebo group actually performed less well after therapy by 1%. Again, the differences between change in the two groups was significant ($p < .02$).

Without question, Hughes' studies have been carefully controlled and executed. They provide strong evidence for the efficacy of the TD therapy.

I now turn to a discussion of the report by Martin et al. (1973) of another independent evaluation of TD therapy. Martin et al. executed a double-blind study including 15 subjects in the experimental group and 8 subjects in the control group. Martin et al. showed that the amount of improvement produced by TD therapy was a function of degree of impairment of hearing. Specifically, there was more improvement in speech discrimination at those levels of speech intensity for which pretherapy scores were relatively low than for those whose pretherapy scores were higher. In particular, when for a given degree of amplitude above SRT the pretherapy speech discrimination scores were at, or better than, 84% there was no significant difference between the improvement of the placebo and the control groups. At amplitudes such that pretherapy scores ranged from 52% to 84%, the experimental group improved 12% while the placebo group only improved 3%. For these levels of intensity the difference between the two groups was significant ($p < .002$). For amplitudes at which pretherapy scores were less than 50%, the experimental group improved 30% while the placebo group improved 11%. Again, for these lower amplitudes, the difference was significant ($p < .024$). Martin et al. concluded "in cases where pre-program scores were 80% or less, our data indicated that electrostimulation improved discrimination and that the improvement was not due to placebo effects."

Thus, what Martin et al. showed was that the slope of the discrimination function steepened more in the experimental group than in the control group. Since one of the significant differences between normals and persons suffering with sensorineural loss is the slope of the discrimination functions they produce, this result was thought to be of potential clinical interest. That is, since normal subjects are characterized by a much steeper discrimination function than are sensorineural impaired subjects, the therapy was thought to be normalizing the hearing ability of sensorneural patients.

It is, however, important to see what Martin and his colleagues did not demonstrate as well as what they did show. While they did show a significant improvement in the slope of the discrimination function as a result of therapy, they did not show precisely the same kind of results as were found by Hughes et al. In particular, what Hughes showed was shift in number of words discriminated at the same objective presentation level. Martin did not find this. What Martin found was a shift in number of words discriminated <u>relative</u> to the SRT. That is, Martin found that the therapy improved the posttherapy discrimination for speech of a given number of decibels above the posttherapy SRT in comparison to the pretherapy discrimination of speech presented the same number of decibels above the pretherapy SRT.

In light of the fact that Martin did not report the sort of changes found by Hughes (1974) or Eckberg (1972) (two authors whose work supported the efficacy of TD therapy), it may be questioned whether the Martin et al. (1973) study should be taken as unambiguously supporting the efficacy of the therapy. On the other hand, it should be noted that examination of the data of Hughes reveals a steepening of the slope of the discrimination function as a result of TD therapy. Hence, it seems likely that Martin, Eckberg and Hughes all observed the same phenomenon. In these early studies, techniques and therapeutic procedures were sufficiently variable to make detailed characterization of the therapeutic effect impossible. What is of primary importance with respect to these studies is that the results of the experimental groups were significantly different from that of the placebo controls along dimensions which would indicate improvement in hearing as a result of therapy.

The third study to be reviewed here is that executed by Eckberg (1972). Eckberg's study involved a rather small number of subjects (6 in the experimental group and 7 in the placebo group). Nevertheless, the average improvement in speech discrimination in the experimental group was so striking (15%) in comparison to the placebo group (1%) that the difference between the two groups was highly significant, $p < .001$.

The fourth set of studies to be considered is that of Gerkin, Glorig, and Roeser (1974). This group executed two experiments to assess the effectiveness of TD therapy. The results of the two experiments were inconsistent. They first ran a pilot study of 10 subjacts which indicated an average (across all presentation levels) improvement of 13% in speech discrimination. In órder to be sure of these results, they executed a subsequent double-blind experiment (8 in the experimental group and 7 in the placebo). The result of the double-blind did not indicate that TD therapy was effective in treatment of sensorineural loss. The experimental group improved 1%, and the placebo group improved 4%, in average (across all presentation levels) speech discrimination.

Gerkin, Glorig and Roeser concluded from their second experiment that TD therapy is ineffective as a treatment for hearing loss. They explained the disparity between their two experiments by arguing that the audiologist who had assessed the subjects' hearing in their first experiment had been biased to hear the subjects improve and had thus misheard the subjects' responses. In the first (pilot) experiment, the subjects had spoken their responses; i.e., they had been asked to attempt to repeat the words presented to them. In the second experiment, the subjects had been instructed to write, rather than speak, their responses. This methodology was thought to avoid the possibility of any "auditor bias".

Gerkin's and his colleagues' conclusion was based on the assumption that the only difference between the two experiments was the method of testing (spoken vs. written responses). Since written responses were less susceptible to experimenter bias (especially in a double-blind context), the latter study seemed to be definitive. This interpretation does, however, strain credulity a bit. The problem is that the amount of improvement in the pilot study (an average of 13% across all levels of amplitude from SRT +0 to SRT +40) is reeally too great to be explained by auditor bias--assuming an experienced and honest clinician. While the effects of tester bias are well known in medical literature (that is the reason for the common use of double-blind procedures), this kind of improvement seems well beyond what an <u>experienced</u> clinician (such as the one involved) could have produced as a result of bias. It seems reasonable to at least look for <u>another</u> difference between the procedures of the two studies which might explain their different results. If no other difference could be found, then we would, perhaps, be forced to accept the interpretation proffered by Gerkin et al.

Interestingly enough, there is another difference to be found between the two studies, and it is a difference which we would have every reason to expect to affect the outcome of the studies. This difference is the current level of the treatment. In order to facilitate the double-blind structure of the experiment, Intellectron Corporation had supplied a switch box through which the current flowed from the current generating machine to the subjects' heads. The setting of the switch determined whether or not a particular subject was receiving therapy. All subjects, active as well as placebo, received "treatment" via the switch box. Measurements made in our laboratory (Prout, 1976) show that even when placed in the active or experimental setting, the switch box cut the current by about 62%. That is, due to an error in the circuitry design, the experimental subjects in Gerkin et al.'s double-blind experiment received about 38% of the current that was given to their pilot group. It seems clear that such a difference in their treatment is at least as plausible an explanation for the differences between the two groups as the conjecture that an experienced audiologist was so convinced of the efficacy of an untried therapy that she misperceived over 10% of her subjects' responses.

In this section I will review the work of Glattke and Simmons (1974) which was aimed at evaluating the efficacy of TD therapy. Glattke and Simmons ran two studies, one which they said to be double-blind and another in which the subjects were all given therapy. That is, the second experiment was not even a single-blind as there was no control group. We will consider the double-blind study first.

The double-blind experiment involved 12 placebo-control and 13 experimental subjects. Subjects received 20 treatments of four per week, for five weeks. They state (p. 94) that "the group mean difference between pre-treatment and post-treatment discrimination scores was never greater than +0.9%, and this positive finding occurred only at SRT + 40dB". They then present the data for level of intensity in relation to SRT (SRT +10dB, SRT + 20dB, SRT +30dB, SRT +40dB). In order to do this, they present four scatterplots of the data, one for each level of intensity. Each plot showed the number of pre-treatment and post-treatment comparisons (re, ears) available for the stimulus presentation level associated with that scatterplot. Pre-treatment scores were shown on the abscissa and post-treatment scores on the ordinate. Each point plotted was said to represent the score obtained prior to and following treatment for one ear. The diagonal (with a slope of 1) defines the no-change limit, and points appearing above the line indicated improvement (that the post-treatment score was greater than the pre-treatment score). It was claimed that "inspection" of the individual panels (scatterplots) makes it apparent that there was no consistent trend for improvement in test scores for individual stimulus levels re: SRT.

Glattke and Simmons tested each subject for SRT and speech discrimination at SRT +10dB, 20dB, 30dB, and 40dB each week, thus allowing for examination of the subjects' performance across the five weeks of therapy. The authors comment on the remarkable variability of the subjects' scores from week to week. They view these fluctuations as giving the false illusions of change due to TD therapy. Inspection of a table showing the week to week progress of both experimental and control subjects at all four levels of stimulus presentation (re.:SRT) reveals only nonsystematic (apparently random) fluctuations of the scores of both groups.

In their group of six subjects run without an accompanying control group, they carried therapy out for 30 sessions of treatment. The discrimination scores of these subjects after 30 treatment sessions were not significantly different from the pre-treatment scores. Thus, in both experiments, the authors failed to find any significant evidence for the efficacy of TD therapy in treating sensorineural hearing loss.

Commenting on their findings, Glattke and Simmons conclude that within-subject variability is responsible for the apparent improvement of certain selected individuals. They suggest that the differences between their findings and those of Hughes, Martin, Eckberg, and Puharich and Lawrence can be accounted for by the fact that written responses (Glattke and Simmons' procedure) are sensitive to variability in a way that spoken responses (the procedure of the other investigators) are not. They argue that "the reduction in variance (brought about by taking spoken responses as opposed to written) may artificially inflate the 'significance' of any group mean differences that are apparent at the outcome of this study". Thus, the suppression of variability resulting from the testing procedure of other workers would be expected to inflate the significance of random fluctuations of the scores of certain subjects. They conclude that "this line of thought seems reasonable enough to prompt a high degree of skepticism in viewing any data gathered using auditory monitoring of repeated measures in sensorineural patients, and we remain unconvinced that Speech Discrimination improvement may be shown under properly controlled evaluation conditions of TD therapy". They then cite the work of Puharich and Lawrence, Martin, and Hughes as exemplary of the sort of work they are not convinced by.

There are a number of dimensions along which the Glattke and Simmons report must be evaluated. I begin with their reporting of their results. In discussing the effects of 20 treatments on speech discrimination, Glattke and Simmons (p. 94) claim that "the group mean differences between pre-treatment and post-treatment discrimination scores was never greater than +0.9% and this positive finding occurred only at SRT +40dB". Now it is a remarkable fact that this statement, which purports to summarize for the reader the effects of TD therapy on group means rather than eccentric individual subjects, appears, if we take their presentation seriously, to be false. Examination of raw data (made available at the AAOO meeting, 1972) indicates, for example, that the experimental group in their souble-blind experiment (26 ears) increased its discrimination at SRT +10dB by an average of approximately 6% per ear. Giving them the benefit of the doubt, however, I assume that their above quoted claim concerns the data from their study of 6 subjects which was run without the benefit of either a double-blind or a control group. Figure 5 in their paper shows that the mean performance of those 6 subjects after 20 treatments had dropped by approximately 5% (out of 100% correct). However, because the number of ears in the active portion of the double-blind was more than twice that in the uncontrolled study, the mean of the combined group could only be brought to less than 0.9% if the decrement in the uncontrolled group was over 10% (more than twice what Glattke and Simmons reported it to be). Thus, it appears that at some point Glattke and Simmons simply (unintentionally, of course) misreported their own data. Unfortunately, I will be forced to show that this kind of disregard for the minimal standards of scientific competence is the rule rather than the exception for their report.

Consider a related example. On page 93, Glattke and Simmons show a set of scatterplots (they label the set Fig.1) which is claimed to represent the changes of the ears in the experimental group. As indicated above, the ordinate corresponds to the post-therapy discrimination score. Thus, a point below the diagonal indicates an ear which scored worse after therapy than before, and a point above the diagonal indicates that the ear scored better after therapy than before. As they have presented the data for 22 ears for SRT +10dB and 20dB, it appears that more ears scored worse after therapy than scored better after therapy. However, the raw data from the double-blind experiment create an opposing impression.

While the scatterplot for SRT +10dB shows at least 14 of 22 ears testing worse after therapy than before, Glattke and SImmons' own raw data for the double-blind experiment shows 14 of 26 ears testing better after therapy than before (3 ears with no change, only 9 ears testing worse after therapy). Their scatterplot for SRT +20dB shows 13 of 22 ears testing worse after therapy than before, with 9 ears improving. However, their raw data show only 11 of 26 ears testing worse after therapy than before, with 14 ears improving. Thus, the scatterplots, while they support the point the authors are trying to argue, are contradicted by the actual trend shown by the experimental subgroups of the double-blind experiment.

This discrepancy between the authors' raw data and the data they report can only be explained if one assumes that the scatterplots represent <u>selected</u> data drawn from the double-blind group <u>and</u> the group which was not run blind or with a control. But then, it is a serious question as to why <u>all</u> the data were not represented in these scatterplots. Furthermore, selection is also involved in their presentation of palcebo data. For example, in the placebo group which contained 24 ears, they report the results of only 8 ears at stimulus level SRT +10dB, 11 ears for SRT +20dB, 17 ears for SRT + 30dB, and 12 ears for SRT +40dB. Glattke and Simmons claim (pg. 94) that "each panel (scatterplot) shows the number of pre-treatment and post-treatment comparisons (ie. ears) that were available for the stimulus presentation level shown in the panel". However, contrary to the authors' claim, since ears are tested for all stimulus levels at the same time, the authors certainly did have access to all the data and <u>could</u> have presented it. On <u>what basis</u> did they decide not to inform the reader about the results of certain ears? Why do they claim to have presented the data which "were available" when it is manifest that other data were available?

Unfortunately, it is not just with the adeqaucy of data presentation that their study runs into trouble. Consider an example. In their raw data they report discrimination data for a certain experimental subject (j.c., right ear) at SRT +10dB. After the first, second, third, fourth, and fifth weeks of therapy, they record that the subject correctly discriminated at levels 68%, 0%, 8%, 80% and 8%, respectively. Preliminary perusal of the data indicates extravagant fluctuation of discrimination scores as well as a before-after difference of -60% discrimination. The data for this ear show considerably worse speech discrimination after therapy than before. Apparently the therapy has had no beneficial effect on hearing, and possibly it has been harmful. However, if one looks at the audiologist's notes at the bottom of the raw data sheet, one notices that different lists of words were used in different testing sessions. In this case, three sets of lists were used. Lists A were used after the first and fourth weeks of therapy, lists B were used after the second and fifth weeks, and lists C after the third week. It is obvious that, even when phonetically balanced, such word lists can differ in difficulty of discrimination, and it is at least possible that such differential difficulty could explain the data under consideration. Suppose that lists A were significantly easier for this subject's right ear to discriminate than lists B. If this were true, then we should not be surprised if the first test (which involved lists A) produced better discrimination than the last test (which involved lists B) <u>even if TD therapy was beneficial to hearing</u>. In the context of a double-blind procedure, the optimal way to determine the effects of therapy would be to compare discrimination scores for the <u>same</u> test-lists.

Another methodological difficulty with Glattke and Simmons' double-blind concerns the authors' failure to administer pre-tests to most of their subjects. They report giving full pre-tests of speech discriminations (testing at 3 or 4 intensities) to only 5 experimental subjects and to only 4 control subjects. To 8 control and 8 experimental subjects, however, they pre-tested at only one level of intensity. For these latter subjects, post-therapy scores had to be compared with test scores obtained <u>after</u> the first week of therapy. Clearly this procedure had the effect of reducing the amount of therapy between the pre- and post-testing from 20 sessions to 16 sessions. It seems equally clear that, if this research had been carefully done, the authors would have taken the trouble to thoroughly pre-test the full 100% (rather than 36%) of the subjects in their double-blind experiment.

I now turn to the question of procedure. It appears that Glattke and Simmons may not have been giving an adequate level of treatment to their subjects. The difficulty stems from the fact that they only began to clean the electrodes through which therapy is administered to the subject "after data has been gathered on 15 subjects" (p. 92). Simmons' original attempt to avoid this criticism was to state in public discussion at the AAOO meeting in Dallas, 1972, that the equipment was a constant current device and thus that this failure to clean the electrodes should in no way be thought to account for his failure to obtain positive results. As it happens, the Intellectron system is <u>not</u> a constant-current device. We have found that a little make-up smeared on the electrodes can cut the actual current across an artificial head with approximately the same electrical properties as a human head by as much as 33%.

Their misunderstanding of the equipment led Glattke and Simmons to cite the stability of the meters as evidence against "the claim that the device could not have been functioning properly on the first (15) subjects". Actually, they are more or less correct in thinking that the current or amperage provided the subjects is correctly indexed by the metering equipment on the machine. However, just because the machine is <u>not</u> a constant current device it must be continually monitored to ensure that it continues to operate at prescribed levels. The authors do not report providing such surveillance.

Moreover, amperage is only one of a number of electronic parameters involved in the therapy. When the electrodes are not clean, current or amperage can only be maintained at prescribed levels by increasing voltage. The effects of different voltages on the therapy are unknown. Further, when the electrodes are not clean, the functional surface area of the electrodes is reduced. In this situation, one is operating with smaller electrodes. But electrode surface area is quite possibly a determiner of current dispersion or density. It seems probable that current dispersion would be an important parameter of the therapy. It is important to note that these facts require not only the cleaning of the electrodes but the cleaning of the skin as well. While Glattke and Simmons report cleaning the electrodes for the last 16 of their 31 subjects, they do not report cleaning the subjects' skin of substances such as oil, perspiration, rouge, powder, etc., which our experience has shown to significantly affect current levels across the head.

Further, it is essential to see that 12 of their 13 experimental double-blind subjects were in that first group of 15 subjects run prior to the cleaning of the electrodes. The electrodes _were_ cleaned for the placebo subjects who were not to receive therapy in any case. The electrodes were _not_ cleaned for 12 of the 13 subjects who received therapy. The confound in this design is obvious. So long as there is as reasonable question as to the result of not cleaning the electrodes, it is impossible to conclude _anything_ from the double-blind study of Glattke and Simmons.

One more point about procedure seems relevant here. Although the original instructions of Puharich and Lawrence claimed 20 treatments to be sufficient to obtain therapeutic results from TD therapy, no other researcher has utilized only 20 treatment sessions. Even prior to Glattke and Simmons' study, both Hughes and Glorig had shown that the therapeutic effect was greater if therapy extended to 30 rather than 20 treatments. Accordingly, Glattke and Simmons' double-blind cannot logically bring into question the positive results of the previously discussed papers (Martin, Hughes, Eckberg). Those researchers _do_ _not_ _claim_ that significant results can be obtained with 20 sessions of therapy.

Moreover, Glattke and Simmons' study of 6 subjects given 30 treatments is, in itself, incapable of shedding light on the problem at hand. That study is flawed by virtue of not being double-blind. As is well known (Rosenthal, 1966), experimenter expectations can influence experimental results _negatively_ as well as positively. No controversial therapy of this sort can legitimately be said to have been evaluated without a double-blind experimental methodology. However, the study under consideration was not even done with a control group (not to mention double-blind). Given the unusual variability of the data, it would be impossible to conclude anything about the efficacy of the TD therapy for these 6 subjects without an associated control group. For the above reasons, it was improper and misleading for Glattke and Simmons to combine the results of the uncontrolled study with those of the active subgroup of the double-blind study when describing the effects of TD therapy. In conclusion, the difficulties accompanying Glattke and Simmons' studies are so great that no competent scientist could think that their failure to show positive results would in any way detract from the significance of the positive results shown by other programs. Those other programs must be evaluated on their own merits. Glattke and Simmons' work is just not comparable to those other studies.

Finally, I wish to comment on the conclusion of Glattke and Simmons that testing procedures involving spoken as opposed to written responses may have artificially suppressed variance and thus inflated the significance of differences observed in studies which show a positive result of TD therapy. First, the spoken response is not necessary for observing improvement as a function of TD therapy. Martin and his colleagues have used written responses exclusively following their first experiment. The results have not changed with the exception of the fact that they are more marked. Second, I have shown that there is good reason to believe that the extreme variability of Glattke and Simmons' data may have resulted from their having used tests of differing levels of difficulty. Lastly, their remarks about the effects of reduced test variability artificially inflating the significance of differences <u>between groups</u> reveals a serious misunderstanding of statistics. Since the studies they are criticizing were run double-blind, there is no possibility that experimenter bias could have preferentially assisted one or another <u>subgroup</u>. Moreover, in those studies the subjects were only tested twice (before and after therapy). Therefore, experimenter bias to suppress variability would be expected to <u>reduce</u>, not enhance, the chances of subjects showing a change as a result of therapy, if such a change occurred. What Glattke and Simmons failed to understand is that any unbiased tendency of the tester to suppress variability would suppress the main effect mean difference as well as the standard deviation of the populations in question. I can only assume that they were acting on incompetent statistical advice in including this argument in their paper. In any case, there is no reason to take their suggestion seriously. It is just another example of the confusion and carelessness which appears to have characterized the conception, execution and reporting of this study. Rather than being scientific, their work represents a kind of play-acting at science. It is totally irresponsible. There is no reason to think that the work of Glattke and Simmons contains any definitive information on the efficacy of TD therapy.

No discussion of these first attempts at evaluating TD therapy would be complete without some comment on the review of Jurgen Tonndorf of these same studies. This is especially true since Tonndorf reached conclusions in direct opposition to those reached by the present reviewer.

The August, 1974, issue of the Archives of Otolaryngology carried three articles--one pro and two con--plus an extended editorial commentary by Jurgen Tonndorf. In his review, Tonndorf surveyed the five published papers on the phenomenon. He claimed that they could be classified into two groups:

1. Those exercising little control and being uncritical in acceptance of results obtained -Puharich and Lawrence, Hughes et al. and Martin et al.

2. Those controlling experimental parameters as well as possible and being more critical toward their own results--Gerkin et al. and Glattke and Simmons.

He continues, "It is probably not a mere coincidence that positive 'treatment' results were reported by the first group and negative ones by the second".

In this context, I will consider the published literature on this subject with a focus on those points used by Tonndorf to establish his position. First, I will discuss the criticism of those studies that have supported transdermal therapy. Then I will point to several of the apparent methodological inadequacies that have been associated with some of the work failing to demonstrate the effectiveness of transdermal therapy. I will show that Tonndorf was mislead because he apparently grossly misunderstood the significance and function of the experimental design and statistical analysis involved in the studies showing positive results.

We will begin with an analysis of Tonndorf's editorial found in the Archives of Otolaryngology, August 1974.

1. Tonndorf notes that the improvements "found (Hughes et al.: 16% to 25% in 35% to 40% of the subjects; and Martin

et al.: 12% (subject number not given)) are not very spectacular".

Several points deserve notice here. First, as is obvious in our presentation, these are PB percentages, not actual percentage improvements. Thus, a subject who improves from PB 50% to PB 70% (i.e., a PB 20% improvement) has actually experienced a 40% improvement in the ability to perceive PB word lists. Second, the Martin et.al. report has been misrepresented. Tonndorf states that "the subject number" was "not given". This is not true. On page 148 we explicitly state that the 12% PB improvement (an 18% improvement) is derived from 14 of 15, or 93% of our subjects. Such an obvious error on Tonndorf's part leads one to ask whether he seriously read the paper.

Actually, the principal point of our presentation of the data was misunderstood by Tonndorf. We were concerned to show that the amount of improvement observed was positively correlated with the degree of pretherapy deficit as indexed by the PB tests. Thus, for 8 of our subjects whose pre-tests for certain levels of amplification averaged about 40%, the improvement was approximately 30% PB (an improvement of 70%) up to a PB score of 70% for those levels of amplification. In general, our findings are in accord with those of Hughes et.al. that the majority of the improvement resulting from this therapy is to be seen in conditions under which the auditory system is being pushed to the limits--for example, under conditions of low amplitude messages and/or competing noise. But these are just conditions under which persons with sensorineural loss suffer most. Therefore, the reported changes, if they index real improvements, may well be of potential clinical significance.

Tonndorf states that "there appears to be uniformity" with respect to electrical current levels used in the various studies. He implies that this fact entails that the method of treatment was the same across the various experiments. Unfortunately, neither the alleged fact nor what it is said to entail are obviously true.

As has already been shown, there is a serious question as to whether the electrodes in Glattke and Simmons' experiment were sufficiently clean to allow for adequate therapy. It is stated that "Hughes et al. found it necessary to modify their technique in their study because of electrode corrosion". He neglects to point out that before Hughes obtained corrosion resistant electrodes, he polished the electrodes weekly in order to remove the current impeding corrosion. This is in contradistinction to Glatte and Simmons who only began to clean their electrodes "after data had been gathered on 15 subjects" (p. 92).

Leaving the issue of the dirty electrodes, we turn to the question of intended current levels. Tonndorf points out that all of the independent investigators followed the manufacturer's instructions concerning current level. He infers that this means that all of the independent investigators used the same current levels. Unfortunately, this is far from being true. Perusal of Hughes' paper (pp. 100, 101), for example, indicates that the manufacturer changed its recommendations at least twice. Which levels were used by which groups?

This is a question which has only recently been answered by Prout (Penn State). Prout has shown that the introduction of the placebo box, supplied by the manufacturer, cut the current drastically. Tonndorf, ignorant of this fact, failed to account for it in comparing experimental results.

Moreover, there appears to have been significant differences in the way in which therapy was monitored. In our work we have always hired a therapist whose responsibility it was to maintain the current levels within a certain preestablished limit continuously throughout the therapy. A number of factors such as head movement, perspiration, and changes in machine operation can alter the current flow during the course of a therapy session. Unfortunately, these details are lacking from the reports of those studies which obtained negative results. They are, however, mentioned and viewed as important by those experimenters who achieved positive results.

Finally, with regard to the general question of whether all experimenters gave the same amount of therapy to their subjects, there is a glaring omission in Tonndorf's account. Tonndorf neglects to report that in the Glattke and Simmons' double-blind study, subjects only received 20 treatments. This is obviously an extremely important point. Moreover, the treatments were given at the rate of four per week instead of the rate of five per week as in other studies mentioned above. Inasmuch as the effect of the therapy appears to be cumulative, this difference in rate of treatment could have been significant also. I find it remarkable that Tonndorf did not note these facts.

Tonndorf goes on to assert that Martin et al. "never questioned the reliability of speech testing". This, also, is not true. Martin et al. were well aware that there is a variability in responding to PB tests, both within and between subjects. Only serious ignorance of inferential statistical procedures could lead Tonndorf to think that we did not take variability into account. Such variability is, of course, accounted for in the statistical test itself. That is the reason for statistics!!

Continuing, Tonndorf touches on the problem of "auditor bias". This is in reference to the explanation proposed by Gerkin et al. for the fact that they observed significant improvements in PB scores after therapy in a pilot study they ran. Gerkin et al. view their positive pilot results as the spurious consequence of "auditor bias" (a bias on the part of the tester which results in the misperception of incorrect responses as correct responses). Of course, their criticism of their own pilot study assumes that auditor bias was not operating as much during the pretest as during the posttest--an assumption which may be to a degree correct. The point is that the only way to know for sure would be to run a control group. This they did not do.

In Tonndorf's statements concerning auditor bias, he suggests that those studies which used spoken rather than written responses were confounded by "auditor bias". He fails to take into account the fact that the experiments of Hughes et al. and Martin et al. were run double-blind. That is, the audiologists did not know which subjects had been in the experimental or in the control groups. Thus, it is impossible, given the nature of double-blind experiments, that "auditor bias" could be invoked to account for postive results. I should have thought that it was universally known that a primary _reason_ for double-blind procedures is to eliminate confounding effects such as "auditor bias".

Tonndorf also takes Hughes to task for running a single-blind experiment. First, it is important to note that Hughes had _already_ run a double-blind experiment which produced positive results. Second, Hughes' single-blind experiment became single-blind only in the sense that the audiologist was able to guess who was in the experimental group because of the subjects' own self-reports of improvement. The audiologist was never told by Hughes who were the active and the placebo subjects. Thus, to the extent that therapy did not affect reports of improvements, Hughes' single-blind experiment remained a double-blind. The experiment can only be said to be single-blind if one assumes, what Tonndorf does not assume, that the therapy creates conditions under which subjects report improvement.

While we are on the topic of control groups, there is a _consistent_ _inconsistency_ in the way Tonndorf interprets experiments not accompanied by a control group. Gerkin et al. reported that they had run a pilot study including 10 subjects. The subjects scored significantly better after therapy than before therapy. Tonndorf uncritically accepted the interpretation proffered by Gerkin et al. that these apparent improvements were a result of "auditor bias" which increased during the therapy presumably because of the audiologist's expectations. Of course, in the absence of a control group, this interpretation is only a speculation. On the other hand, Glattke and Simmons ran an uncontrolled study including six subjects. They did not achieve significant improvement. In this case, Tonndorf opted to believe these results in the absence of a control group. This is somewhat surprising since the variance of the data Glattke and Simmons reported was remarkably high. Therefore, any interpretations of such data would require a placebo--double-blind contol group. But then, if one considers the general incompetence of Tonndorf's above mentioned remarks relating to test variability and "auditor bias" perhaps it is not so surprising.

Tonndorf goes on to suggest that what is require is some sort of evidence of cochlear change as a result of the TD therapy. He states, for example, that a shift in SRT scores would constitute such evidence. As will be shown below, more careful investigations have shown such a shift in SRT. Further, there is other work which will be discussed that gives both empirical and theoretical reasons for believing that TD therapy affects cochlear change.

In summary, Tonndorf's conclusions are not supported by careful analysis of the papers under discussion. It seems undoubtable that a more careful reading of those papers and an elementary understanding of experimental and statistical methodology would have dissuaded Tonndorf from coming to the conclusions that he did.

In this section, I will summarize the procedures and related findings of the five double-blind studies intended to replicate the original Puharich and Lawrence experiment. There are significant differences ampong protocols as well as the findings of these studies. I will show that the differences in results reported by various groups correlate in a meaningful way with the differences among protocol used by these groups. The dimensions of difference are as follows:

A. Amount of therapy--The amount of therapy given to subjects by various experimenters varied. Certainly, these differences must be considered in evaluating the different results reported by those experiments.

    1. Number of hours of treatment--Four or five studies involved 30 hours of treatment. One study involved 20 hours of treatment. The study using 20 hours of therapy did not report improvement as a result of therapy. Three of the four studies using 30 hours of therapy did report a positive therapeutic effect.

    2. Cleaning of electrodes and skin--Insofar as clean electrodes and skin are required for optimal conductivity, it is reasonable to think that those groups who cleaned the

electrodes and skin of their experimental subjects would be giving a greater amount of therapy than those who did not. Four groups reported such cleaning; three of them observed improvement in their subjects. The one group which did not clean the electodes for its experimental subjects observed no therapeutic effect.

3. Current levels-- Reports of exact (numerical values) current levels are conspicuously absent from the two negative papers. It is thus not clear what current levels their subjects received. On the other hand, two of the three positive reports indicated using current levels with numerical value at or above those recommended by the manufacturer.

B. Methods of Assessment-- The three papers reporting therapeutic effect utilized spoken subjects' responses. The two groups not reporting therapeutic effect utilized written responses. If these experiments had not been double-blind, then this factor would justifiably influence our interpretation of the reported results. However, since they were all run double-blind, there is no reason to think that this factor could have influenced the results, one way or the other. The suggestion by Glattke and Simmons to the contrary is a conceptual error.

D. Experimental Design-- There were differences in experimental design, and such differences must always be considered when evaluating differential experimental results.

1. Randomization of subject assignment-- In a double-blind experiment, it is essential that the order of treatment and testing be either random or balanced. This insures that the two groups (experimental and control) are exposed to essentially the same conditions. Three of the four experiments run in this way produced positive results. The study not run in this fashion (Glattke and Simmons) failed to show results.

2. Difficulty of pre- and posttesting-- In order to determine the effect of TD therapy on speech perception, it is essential the pretest be the same (or be known to be of the same difficulty) as the posttest. Of the four studies using well known tests, three showed positive results. Glattke and Simmons' study which involved a relatively unknown "in house" test, failed to meet this condition and, failed to obtain any results.

E. Evidence of Investigator Concern-- One of the studies reporting negative results was rendered valueless due to apparent carelessness in the collection and reporting of data. I do not suggest that adequate subject testing and presentation of data would have resulted in a positive finding. I do claim that failure to pretest and that careless and misleading reporting of data are, from the scientific viewpoint, intolerable. They are also, I think, plausible indeces as to the degree to which Glattke and Simmons were serious about investigating the matter at hand. There is little reason to take the study of Glattke and Simmons as an example of serious scientific work.

F. Summary-- It is reasonable to assume that differences in protocol were, in large measure, responsible for the differences in reported results. In general, those experiments in which subjects were given more therapy, and better surveillance, tended to give better results. Also, those experiments which were more carefully designed tended to show more therapeutic effect.

I have here demonstrated that the arguments presented by Tonndorf and Glattke and Simmons in support of their conclusions have been characterized by both negligence and incompetence. For this reason authors who wish to spare themselves public embarrassment should avoid uncritical citation of the work of Glattke and Simmons, and Tonndorf. In an attempt to summarize the literature for practicing physicians, Bess, Schwartz, Seestedt and McConnell (1975, in Pediatrics) erred by depending unquestioningly on the analysis of Tonndorf. Their review is thus flawed with the inadequacies associated with Tonndorf's paper. However, not content with that, they add a measure of their own. They show no evidence of having carefully read the primary literature. Thus, for example, in their Table III they grossly distort the work of Hughes in several significant wasys. First they report falsely that Hughes' subjects received only 20 treatments. His paper clearly states that he administered 30 treatments. Second, they report falsely that Hughes only ran 16 subjects. Again, his report clearly states that 47 subjects participated in his two blind studies.

Messers. Bess, Schwartz, Seestedt, and McConnell owe a public apology to Hughes, Martin and the readers of Pediatrics who had a right to assume that those authors would take the trouble to read the papers they were reviewing. To assume that misrepresentation of a scientific paper will be condoned by the scientific community simply because that paper espouses an unpopular position would be to seriously underestimate the intellectual honesty of the members of that community. Past and potential contributors to the literature in the area should understand that such pseudo-scholarly irresponsibility will be exposed.

In this section, I will describe studies which have not been directly aimed at replicating the original Puharich and Lawrence experiment. Most of these studies (the work done at U.S.C. and Penn State) presuppose the efficacy of the therapy.

They are not aimed at showing that Puharich and Lawrence's work can be replicated. These investigators (Martin & Hughes) have already accomplished such replications. Thus, for the last several years, the P.S.U. and U.S.C. groups have concentrated on determining the parameters of successful therapy. During that time, they have had intensive and often repeated experience with almost 300 subjects. The result is that when their later findings are combined with their original research, it is possible to begin to characterize the conditions required for successful therapy.

I now summarize the work of Hughes and his colleagues at U.S.C. Hughes has looked at TD therapy in the context of a number of different subject characteristics and protocol variations. These variations (subsequently to be described) were variations of a more or less standard protocol which had emerged from the original double-blind studies. I begin by describing that standard protocol.

Evaluation methods consisted of three parts. First, pure tone audiograms. Second, speech reception thresholds (SRT). Third, discrimination functions (W-22 PB word lists) at sensation levels of SRT + 10, 20 and 30 dB. The same lists and word delivery intensity levels were used in the same sequence after therapy as before. Starting scores of 82% or greater were not accepted.

According to Hughes, Arthur, and Whittaker (1974), the standard protocol of procedure has been as follows:
    a. Binaural, sensorineural impaired subjects;
    b. Evaluated twice, with several days between, before and after the procedure using sensation levels of 10, 20, and 30dB above SRT, and for most, at the sensation level of 20dB with 7 and 0 S/N ratios of white noise;
    c. The difference between scores taken before and after was entered only if starting score was below 82%;
    d. Electrostimulation with seven modes of equal length was given 30 times, 5 days a week, for 49 minutes per day, at 2.5 - 3.5 ma in modes 1 and 2 and 15 - 20 ma in modes 3 -7;
    e. Supervision was always provided; and
    f. Skin and electrodes were cleaned thoroughly with isopropanol before and sometimes during treatment.

The effects of selected deviations from this protocol were determined with 12 groups. The subjects were randomly chosen sensorineural impaired patients of Los Angeles County-U.S.C. Medical Center. None with a stapes replacement or Meniere's disease was used (pp. 2,3,4).

The results show:
    1. No difference in percentage improvement as between mild (<50dB) and moderate-severe sensorneural loss. Two

groups (N = 27 and 17) mild loss improved 15% and 13%, respectively. One group of moderate-to-severe loss (N = 26) showed a mean gain of 12.5%.

2. Persons over 77 years old (N = 27) showed a mean improvement of 5.4%. A comparable group between 18-78 years of age (N = 26) gained 12.5%. A group of high school students (N = 14) also with comparable hearing loss averaged 12.5% improvement. Thus, the therapeutic effect was markedly reduced for aged subjects. However, Hughes reports that experience with individual subjects suggests that "total health may be a more important criterion than age upon which to select subjects in the older age brackets".

3. A group of persons with severe sensorineural loss in only one ear showed a gain of only 2.2%. This fact suggests a link between certain etiologies and responsiveness to therapy.

4. TD therapy used in conjunction with niacin showed no synergy. There was a gain of 11.3%. Papaverine, on the other hand, appeared to negatively interact with TD therapy. A group (N = 12) receiving papaverine along with therapy showed an average gain of only 5.3%.

5. A group of 13 subjects received therapy at a current level of about 65% of that used by Hughes in other studies. This level of treatment was enforced by a machine with a cutoff supplied by the manufacturer. Interestingly, the same equipment was supplied to Gerkin et al. for their double-blind and to Glattke and Simmons for their second experiment. The average improvement for this group was 8.7%. This improvement is considerably less than that normally achieved by Hughes. These data must certainly affect our interpretation of the data reported by both Gerkin et al. and Glattke and Simmons. Even Hughes, who supports the efficacy of TD therapy, cannot obtain positive results using the current levels Gerkin et al. and Glattke and Simmons were using.

6. Hughes tried giving 98 minutes (as opposed to 49 minutes) of therapy for 15 days (as opposed to 30 days). The result for 15 subjects was an average improvement of 7.3%. This indicates that the change the therapy produces takes a minimal amount of time as might be expected of certain neurocellular changes. Hughes also attempted therapy using only the bare electrodes (2 of the 6 modes normally programmed into therapy). The result for 13 subjects was an average improvement of 11%.

7. Subjects tested in white noise background showed somewhat more improvement (14%) when tested in quiet background.

Several points emerge as a result of an overall look at

Hughes' work. First, Hughes has explored the parameters of
the TD therapy with more than 180 subjects (not including
those subjects involved in his first three experimental as-
sessments of the therapy reported in a previous section).
This program of research is in impressive contrast to the
less than 40 subjects which is the total number of subjects
given the therapy by both the Callier and Stanford groups
combined. Second, the mean improvements of the experimental
groups is clearly well beyond the average 3.5% improvements
of all the placebo groups run in relation to the therapy.
Third, when Hughes used machines which delivered the same current as those used by Gerkin et al. in their double-blind and
Glattke and Simmons in their second (uncontrolled experiment),
Hughes could not get results either. This indicates that the
failure of these investigators to find positive results can
be largely attributed to the low level of current being delivered to their subjects.

In this section, I discuss the work of Brooks and Harrison (1974). Brooks and Harrison did not attempt a replica-
tion of the original work of Puharich and Lawrence. Instead,
they chose to assess the effectiveness of the TD therapy in
facilitating speech perception in situations more "real-life"
in character than the PB word tests. In order to do this,
they adopted Jerger's Synthetic Sentence Identification procedure (SSI).

In this procedure (SSI), the subject is given a sheet of
paper on which are printed 10 pseudo-sentences (approxima-
tions to English). These pseudo-sentences, while not being
fully grammatical, possess a number of the constraints of ordinary English sentences. These pseudo-sentences are presented, one at a time, in random sequence. Each pseudo-sentence
is presented three times; thus, the subject receives 30
pseudo-sentences for any one level of presentation. At the
same time the pseudo-sentences are being presented, the subject is also being presented background masking which consists
of a male voice reading a story about Davy Crockett. The subject's task is to identify which pseudo-sentence is presented
as each one is given. Thirty correct identifications would
be scored as 100%.

It is clear that, in a number of ways, the SSI approximates those situations in which persons with sensorineural
loss have the most difficulty (situations in which several
persons are talking at the same time). Nevertheless, it is
important to understand that Jerger and his colleagues designed the SSI in order to diagnose serious retro-cochlear
lesions rather than sensorineural disorders. In fact, Jerger
himself recommended to Hughes (personal communication) that
the SSI not be used to evaluate the standard population with

sensorineural loss. The SSI is not sensitive to high frequency loss such as is typical in sensorineural loss. What is important for our purposes here is to understand that the results of the SSI do not correlate well with those obtained fron PB lists, especially in the case of subjects with sensorineural loss (Jerger & Thelin, 1968; Nelson, 1968). Thus, while the SSI may test an important dimension of sensorineural hearing loss, it is quite probably not the same dimension as is tested by the PB word lists. For example, Martin has shown the TD therapy to improve speech perception as measured by the SSI in subjects for whom the TD therapy did not improve discrimination as measured by PB word lists. Accordingly, it is apparent that the results of a study like that by Brooks and Harrison cannot reflect directly on the question of the replicability of the original Puharich and Lawrence study.

Brooks and Harrison executed a double-blind experiment in which subjects were tested with the SSI at 30dB above SRT (as estimated by pure tone averages). They ran five conditions of masking: One in which there was not competing signal, and four masking conditions in which the signal-to-noise ratios were +10, 0, -10, and -20. The differences between the improvement of the experimental and placebo groups were +1.54%, +8.25%, -.83%, +1.46%, and -3.72%, respectively. As a whole, there was no difference between the changes in the experimental and control groups. Inspection of the data increases a superiority (8.25%) of the experimental over the control group in only that case in which S/N = +10.

Some of these apparently negative findings can be explained if one considers data collected in our laboratory also using the SSI as the dependent measure. In the absence of competing noise, the level of presentation of the to-be-perceived stimulus (approximately SRT +30dB) is typically too high to allow observation of improvement. At this presentation level, we were not able to discover a therapeutic effect because the pretherapy scores (usually well above 90%) were so close to being 100% that there was no possibility of measuring any therapy-induced improvement.

Moreover, the Penn State group has used the SSI holding the to-be-detected signal at 60dB SPL (probably quite close to SRT +30dB for many persons with sensorineural loss). The signal-to-noise ratio has been swept from -30dB to +30dB in steps of 6dB. We have also held the signal-to-noise ratio equal to zero and swept the signal from 0dB to 90dB. For both of these conditions we have found strikingly significant differences between the experimental and placebo control groups. Thus, we have not been able to replicate Brooks and Harrison's failure to find effects of the TD therapy on speech discrimination as measured by the SSI (see Tables 1 and 2).

Martin and his colleagues have been engaged in examining the TD therapy since 1969. During that time, they have run a number of studies involving 80 subjects. The results of these studies gives a more elaborate picture of the results of TD therapy and of the parameters which make for successful therapy.

In particular, the Penn State group has further demonstrated the principle that the therapeutic effects of TD therapy are most evident in cases where the to-be-detected signals are close to threshold and subject to masking. That is, they have shown that, in contexts most like everday life, subjects improve most. Second, they have explored the character of the change produced by the therapy. These results indicate the possibility of cochlear changes resulting from the therapy. Third, from their own work, and analysis of the work of other groups, they have shown the systematic correlation between the amount of current given during therapy and the amount of therapeutic effect. This correlation explains nicely the failure of some investigators to obtain results. Fourth, they have developed data which support a conception of the psychophysical function of the therapy. That is, they have proposed a mechanism on the psychophysiological level which accounts for much of the data we now have on the effects of this TD therapy.

(1) Everyday speech is variously estimated as being of from 40 to 60dB SPL in intensity. Thus, persons with sensorineural hearing loss usually have sufficiently high SRT's that the great majority of everyday communications goes on at a level of not more than 20dB above SRT. In fact, it is not unusual for such persons to have an SRT in the range of 40 to 60db. Hence, improvements in discrimination at SRT +20, 10 and even 0dB can have great social benefit for many of these people. Accordingly, it has been encouraging to observe that the most significant improvement produced by the therapy occurs at SRT +10 and 20dB. Martin and his colleagues explored this possbility further by taking discrimination scores at SRT +0 as well as SRT +10, 20, 30 and 40dB.

In every case when a group showed improvement as a result of TD therapy, the greatest change was observed for presentation levels of SRT +0dB. Consider, three such groups in which PB discrimination measures were taken. These contained 9, 14, and 9 subjects. The improvement at SRT +0dB as opposed to SRT + 10dB for these groups was 48% as opposed to 24%, 17% as opposed to 6%, and 28% as opposed to 14%, respectively. In our experience, the percentage improvement at SRT +0dB is often twice the improvement at SRT + 10dB.

Not only is this finding promising in relation to the question of the social benefit of TD therapy, it helps to explain certain incongruities in the literature. For example Hughes reports having no success with the modified rhyme test. This is a test in which the subject is shown a set of typed words which rhyme. He is then aurally presented one of these words. Hughes presented the to-be-recognized words to his subjects at the recommended intensity of 30dB above SRT. On the other hand, using this test we have shown in one group (N = 9) a highly significant average improvement of 27% at SRT + 0dB. It is clearly possible that Hughes did not obtain results because his testing level was too high.

Finally, by using the SSI materials, Martin et al. have demonstrated (Tables 1 and 2) a significant improvement in percentage of items perceived. The optimum difference (significant, $p < .05$, Mann-Whitney U-test) between the means of the placebo and experimental groups was 34%. What is all the more remarkable about these results is that the shift in PB word scores for these same subjects is not significant. Accordingly, we have supported Hughes' contention that some subjects can report social benefits from the therapy and show little or no improvement in PB discrimination scores. The SSI materials do form a fairly good analogue to the sort of social situation in which persons suffering from sensorineural loss report the greatest difficulties. Used properly (at sufficiently low intensities), the SSI can be a very useful tool for demonstrating the effectiveness of TD therapy at improving speech perception in everyday settings.

(2) The character of the change produced by the therapy has not been clear from the beginning. The first reports of Hughes, Martin and Eckberg indicated no change in SRT. However, subsequent work by Martin has shown some change in SRT as a function of TD therapy. Early reports that the SRT did not shift probably resulted from testing SRT at 5dB intervals instead of 2dB intervals (which have been used subsequent to our first double-blind). By testing at 5dB intervals, many changes in SRT were probably missed which have subsequently been detected by testing at 2dB intervals. Improvement in PB discrimination scores now appears to be correlated with improvement in SRT. We have observed group mean shifts in SRT of as much as 10dB. Note that the shift in SRT is consistent, as Tonndorf admits, with the view that the therapy produces changes in the cochlea.

Another significant discovery has been that discrimination scores may continue to improve for several months after therapy. Thus, one group, (N = 14) showed a quite significant difference between pretherapy and posttherapy testing.

Table 1. The affects of TD therapy as measured by the SSI, holding S/N=0 and varying signal level.

		-25	-20	-15	-10	-5	Base	+5	+10	+15	+20
Experimental Group, (N=10), Average Percent Correct	Pretest	0	0	0	0	0	24	47.5	64	73	77
	Posttest	0	1.5	3.5	16.5	36	60.5	80	89.5	89.5	89.5
	Posttest minus Pretest	0	1.5	3.5	16.5	36	35.5	32.5	25.5	16.5	12.5
Placebo Group, (N=6), Average Percent Correct	Pretest	0	0	0	0	0	23.5	61.5	77.5	86.5	89
	Posttest	0	0	0	3	15	42.5	60.5	74	82.5	87.5
	Posttest minus Pretest	0	0	0	13	15	19	-1	-3.5	-4	-1.5
Changes in Experimental Group minus change in the Placebo Group		0	1.5	3.5	3.5	21	16.5	33.5	29	20.5	14

Amplitude of Presentation in dB (normalized)

Table 2. The effects of TD therapy as measured by the SSI, holding message at 60dB and varying S/N.

		S/N in dB (normalized)							
		-18	-12	-6	Base	+6	+12	+18	+24
Experimental Group, (N=10), Average Percent Correct	Pretest	0	0	0	16	42	73.5	87.5	91
	Posttest	0	4.25	22.5	49	73.5	92	97	98.5
	Posttest minus Pretest	0	4.25	22.5	33	31.5	18.5	9.5	7.5
Placebo Group (N=6) Average Percent Correct	Pretest	0	0	0	22.5	49.5	72	81.5	93
	Posttest	0	0	5.5	21	55.5	72	80.5	93
	Posttest minus Pretest	0	0	5.5	-1.5	6	0	-1.0	0
Change in Experimental Group minus change in the Placebo Group		0	4.25	17	34.5	25.5	18.5	10.5	7.5

63

When this group was tested at SRT + 10dB one and two months after the therapy had been discontinued, there was an improvement of about 6% (PB scores) beyond the posttherapy assessment. After three and one-half months, the scores all returned to pretherapy levels.

(3) In examining the electronics of the TD devices, Prout (1976) discovered that the manufacturer-supplied switch used in all placebo experiments cut the current as much as 62%. This fact can, of course, explain some of the difficulty early researchers had in obtaining significant results in double-blind studies. Prout then considered all of the then available work in order to explore the relationship between amount of current given during therapy and the amount of therapeutic results obtained.

His findings show a systematic positive correlation between amount of current and amount of therapeutic effect. This kind of variation of the parameters which affect therapeutic results is a most impressive demonstration that the therapy is efficacious.

(4) At this juncture, I consider the theory proposed by Michael and Bienvenue (1976) of Penn State as to the character of sensorineural hearing loss. This theory explains many hitherto unintegrated facts concerning hearing loss. Moreover, on the assumption that TD therapy ameliorates sensorineural hearing loss, a number of the effects of the therapy noted above can be explained in terms of this theory. The theory thus provides a partial rationale for the efficacy of the TD therapy.

Their theory is grounded on the notion of the "critical band". "The critical band may be defined as some frequency bandwidth beyond which a listener's subjective response will change, i.e., the loudness sensation produced by any random noise with a bandwidth less than that of the critical band will appear to remain constant with bandwidth changes if the sound pressure level is held constant. However, as the bandwidth is increased beyond that of the critical band, for the same sound pressure level, the loudness sensation increases.

Critical bands are too narrow and sharply defined in frequency limits to be explained solely by the mechanical vibration characteristics of the inner ear structures (Von Bekesy, 1960,1962). Thus, the mechanical tuning of the inner ear must be sharpened by a neural, inhibitory network. In this model of the cochlea, the sensation region corresponding to one critical band is surrounded by a region where there is mechanical stimulation, but response to this stimulation is neurally inhibited. In effect, there is a limit to the amount of neural units within the inner ear that can respond to a sound having a given frequency range. The mechanisms for such an inhibiting phenomenon is a network of inhibitory neurons that serves to cut off sensory response to sound in the frequency range outside the critical band region.

The distribution of inhibitory neurons within the cochlea is primarily in the region of outer hair cells while the components of the auditory nerve carrying sensory messages up to the brain are primarily within the inner hair cells, (Spoendlin, 1973). High level noise exposure is known to cause structural damage to the outer hair cell region of the cochlea before the injury invades the inner hair cell region, (Paparella and Melnik, 1967), and thus, due to their location and innervation patterns, the inhibitory neurons. It is proposed, therefore, that the early stages of noise exposure may result in a condition such that neural pathways to higher auditory centers remain relatively intact, but inhibitory pathways are damaged. In such a case, wider than normal critical bands would be expected. In fact, several studies have indicated that injury to the inner ear does result in widening of critical bands, (DeBoer, 1961, Sharf and Hellinan, 1960, Jerger, Burney and Grump, 1974). The widening of critical bands would result in a greater number of sensory transducers being made available for responding to input in a given frequency region. Thus, widened critical bands would give rise to an abnormally rapid growth in loudness perception; that is, recruitment. Support for the contention that widening of critical bands precedes the loss in threshold sensitivity comes from Bekesy (1960b). He reported that listeners exposed to high level sound showed a permanent decrease in their difference limen (i.e. recruitment) but **only** temporary (15-minute) threshold loss for pure tones. That is, in these cases, recruitment preceded the development of pure tone hearing threshold loss.

Distortion of sound signals caused by widening of the critical bands along with loudness recruitment may explain several parameters of cochlear hearing loss that are not well understood at this time. Persons with cochlear hearing loss typically demonstrate difficulty in pitch discrimination tasks. This would be a predicted result of the loss of the fine tuning within the cochlea due to widening of critical bands. Cochlear hearing loss is also accompanied by poor speech discrimination ability. This is the commonly reported experience of being able to hear speech but being unable to understand it. Since discrimination is dependent to some extent upon pitch discrimination, a loss in speech discrimination is to be expected in an ear that has lost inhibitory neurons.

This theory also lends itself well in explaining the particular difficulty that a person with a noise-induced hearing loss has in communicating in a noisy environment since more masking noise would be sensed by an ear with a widened critical band. Within the framework of this theory, the disruption of speech discrimination ability is dependent upon a process that is relatively independent of hearing threshold acuity. Since the widening of critical bands is due to cochlear changes that do not require changes in the neural input to the auditory nerve, speech or pitch discrimination may be independent of hearing threshold loss. The value of the model suggested above is clear when one considers that it has long been recognized that hearing thresholds are a poor predictor of speech discrimination ability" (pp. 53, 54).

The significance of this theory for our understanding of the effect of the TD therapy is twofold. First, it allows us to explain a number of the changes the therapy produces. Second, it gives us some clues as to possible physiological locus of the therapeutic effect.

One of the most stable findings has been that TD therapy improves detection of speech in noise more than detection in quiet background. Moreover, it has been shown that the detection of speech itself is improved more than the detection of pure tones. Further, as we have seen, there is more improvement in the detection of speech which is close to threshold intensities than that which is well above threshold. It is plausible to think that these three facts are really the result of the same sort of physiological change. Speech, for example, contains considerable broad-band noise along with the cues which allow it to be discriminated. Hence, even in a quiet background, speech is accompanied by noise in a way that pure tones are not. Also, speech lies close to threshold intensity (even when presented in quiet background) necessarily involves the listener being confronted with a lower signal-to-noise ratio than when the speech is presented at well above threshold intensities.

According to Michael and Bienvenue, widened critical bands wouls permit more extraneous noise to be confused with the signal and thus would produce a deficit of signal detection in noise background. On the assumption that TD therapy acts to decrease the critical band which has been pathologically widened by environmental noise or other stress to the outer hair cells of the cochlea and their associated neural structures, we would expect improved detection of signals in noisy backgrounds. Accordingly, we would expect more improvement in the detection of speech in noise than in the detection of speech in quiet background, and in the detection of speech close to threshold intensities than in the detection of speech well above those intensities.

We would also expect the perception of pure tones in

noise to be facilitated by TD therapy. Such results have been obtained in Kohut (1977). Working under the direction of Dr. Bienvenue, Kohut has shown a shift in the amount of noise required to mask pure tones as a function of TD therapy. For eight persons with sensorineural loss, Kohut has shown that TD therapy increases the amplitude necessary to mask a 2000 Hz tone (presented at 5dB SL) by about 15dB. Thus, it is quite possible to show that TD therapy shifts the thresholds of pure tones if they are accompanied by masking. Not only this, but by varying the frequency of the masking tone it appears to be possible to obtain information about critical bands. The data are consistent with the hypothesis that TD therapy produces a narrowing of critical band width. In a subsequent section, we will consider the evidence for cochlear change from the standpoint of physiological parameters.

This section I recount the clinical work done at Intellectron Corporation. This work is in no way experimental, yet it is informative from a clinical point of view. No account of the TD therapy would be complete without some mention of it. There are two aspects to this work. First, a number of physicians in the New York City area have referred their patients to Intellectron for treatment. These patients are then given 30 treatments at the Intellectron Corporation offices. In most cases, Intellectron does not test the patient. The patient is tested before and after therapy by the referring agency or by some other independent agency. Thus, the changes noted in these patients are of the sort that might be expected to be observed in clinical practice.

In this report, I will only be concerned with those patients who were tested <u>exclusively</u> by persons <u>not</u> associated with Intellectron. Also, I have not included in my analysis any ears which began with a discrimination score of 0% and did not improve. Such ears are, quite possibly, profoundly deaf and thus not appropriate for the therapy. The only other restriction I made was to eliminate any ears for which the initial discrimination score was greater than 80%. Given these limits, I simply averaged the changes for both ears for the lowest recorded presentation level. Of the 55 subjects who had at least one ear that met the above conditions, the mean improvement was 17% (of a perfect 100% correct). Clinically, this seems to be quite good.

In this section, I summarize the most important results of the studies discussed above--studies not intended to replicate Puharich and Lawrence, but to explore TD therapy along other dimensions. First, there is overwhelming evidence that TD therapy improves discrimination of signals presented in some noise more than signals presented with minimal competition. Even pure tone perception, which has been generally thought to be unaffected by TD therapy, was facilitated when the pure tones were presented along with a masker. This finding is consistent with a hypothesis about the general nature of sensorineural loss. If that hypothesis is correct, and if TD therapy mitigates sensorineural loss, then the locus of the effect of TD therapy is cochlear (possibly involving the hair cells and related neural structures).

Second, the changes brought about by the therapy require a minimal amount of time (more than 15 days). However, once it has been established, improvement may actually continue to increase for as long as 3 months after therapy. Together, these facts indicate that the therapy produces relatively long-term and stable changes (probably in cochlear and retrocochlear metabolism). Further evidence for the thesis that the therapy affects metabolically-based dysfunctions is found in the lack of improvement Hughes noted for patients with severe loss in only one ear. In such cases, general metabolic dysfunction seems not to be so likely (otherwise we would expect some loss in both ears). Therefore, if TD therapy facilitates the metabolism of subfunctional cochlear (possibly even retrocochlear) cells, we would not predict it to be beneficial in such cases.

Third, there is now considerable evidence relating the degree of effect to the amount of current delivered during therapy. Not only does this fact serve to explain the negative results of early investigators, it provides important evidence that the therapy is responsible for the observed changes in perceptual capacity. The fact that different levels of current produce different results is a demonstration that the therapeutic current is an efficacious parameter in affecting changes in perceptual capacity.

Fourth, as we move toward testing situations which are more analogous to "real-life" contexts, we find improvement even more marked than the PB tests indicated. Improvement in speech perception is greatest in those situations in which the speech is either presented at low intensities or masked. Using the SSI, for example, improvements are observed in the range of from 30% to 40%, even for subjects who show little or no improvement on PB word tests. These facts support the potential clinical value of the therapy.

We now turn to the question of the physiological effect of the TD therapy. As we have seen, the rationale of the therapy has been developed around a conception of the nature of sensorineural loss. On this theory, damage to the outer hair cells and/or the neural structures wuth which they are associated results in a widening of critical bands. Thus, the ear, not being able to separate information from the noise which falls within the critical band, becomes progressively less able to detect signals in noise background. This theory is supported by a good deal of physiological as well as psychophysical data. Moreover, examination of the sorts of changes produced by TD therapy shows that, in every case, improvement is most evident for signals which are to some degree masked by noise. In fact, Kohut (working at Penn State) has shown that even the threshold for pure tones can be improved by TD therapy if those tones are partially masked. Further, the pattern of masking resulting from the relationship between the frequency of the masker and the masked tone indicates a narrowing of the critical band as a result of TD therapy.

Accordingly, we have given, at the psychophysical level, a rationale for the efficacy of the therapy. It remains to be shown that the TD therapy could plausibly be thought to have a positive influence on the cochlea. In particular, it must be shown that it is reasonsble to think that TD therapy is beneficial to the hair cells and/or the neural structures associated with them. If this can be done, and I think that it can, then a coherent rationale for the procedure will have been given. Although there are a number of intriguing scientific questions left to be answered (there always are), there is good reason to believe that we can at this time approach identifying the physiological locus of the effect.

The first point to be made is that it may be meaningful to speak of the possibility of beneficially affecting the hair cells and their associated neural structures. If hearing loss were only a result of cell death, then no therapy could be expected to be beneficial. The reason is simply that cell replacement is impossible for the systems in question. However, there is no reason to believe that sensorineural loss is solely a result of cell death. It is not implausible that cells might go through a prolonged period of sub- or nonfunctionality prior to the onset of irreversible structural changes resulting in death. Accordingly, if such cells could be made functional again, one would expect an improvement in hearing. Moreover, it would be predicted that the degenerative processes in the cochlear and retrocochlear systems could be slowed down.

Second, there is evidence to show that we might expect TD therapy to facilitate the metabolism for such sub- or nonfunctional cells. There are two well-demonstrated physiological effects of TD therapy. First, Puharich and Lawrence have shown that when placed in an electric field like the one involved in TD therapy, blood cells will stand apart from one another and from the walls of their container. Clearly, the field is producing a charge on the blood cell membranes. Now, it is known that a number of different stresses can reduce membrane potentials for many kinds of cells. Moreover, membrane potentials are certainly important for cell metabolism (ion exchange, etc.). If it is hypothesized that cells in the cochlea respond to stress by lowered membrane potential and that such a change renders them subfunctional, then an agent which would repolarize their membranes might be expected to increase their level of functioning. It is at least possible that TD therapy does just this. It is possible that TD therapy, by placing a charge on cell membranes, has the effect of repolarizing them. It is interesting to recall in this connection that Martin and Prout have shown the therapeutic effect to continue to improve <u>after therapy has been discontinued</u>. Apparently, the therapy initiates physiological changes which continue, for a while, to regenerate cell metabolism.

Third, Hughes has recently shown that TD therapy decreases surface circulation and thus improves <u>deep</u> circulation and, hence, possibly facilitates metabolism in the deeply placed auditory mechanism. In general, blood circulation is notoriously decreased in the population most prone to sensorineural hearing loss.

Now, the suggestions made above are plausible but still hypothetical. They show how TD therapy <u>might</u> beneficially affect the hair cells and their associated neural structures. What is required in order to adequately support the rationale for TD therapy developed here, however, is <u>direct</u> evidence that TD therapy <u>does</u> beneficially affect those parts of the auditory system. Fortunately, we now have such evidence. Bochenek and Bochenek (1976) have shown that VIII nerve action potential responses to broadband clicks increase as a function of TD therapy. That is, they treated 16 persons with sensorineural loss with TD therapy. On electrocochleagraphic recordings made after TD therapy, a positive response to a click of lower intensity than that required for such a response before therapy was found for 7 patients. Examination of their data shows a drop in threshold and an increased amplitude of action potentials to clicks above threshold. No subjects got worse. Moreover, the shift in physiological threshold was accompanied by a shift in psychophysical threshold (personal communication with the authors).

There are several important facts to be noted here. First, this action potential is a response which is relatively independent of "psychological" factors. For example, it can be obtained while the patient is asleep. Second, amplitude of the action potential is well known to be causally connected with psychophysical threshold. Third, the hair cells and related neural structures are known to be implicated in the production of the VIII nerve action potential.

There is, therfore, now no question that TD therapy affects the hearing mechanism in a way which would be expected to produce improved hearing. Further, the locus of the effect implicates the hair cells and their associated neural structures. This fact supports the critical band theory proposed above. There can now be no doubt that TD therapy produces cochlear effects which are directly correlated with the ability to hear.

Conclusion

In conclusion, the significance of the findings of Bochenek and Bochenek cannot be overemphasized. The original disbelief which confronted the report by Puharich and Lawrence stemmed primarily from the fact that there was no coherent explanation for their results. It is now possible to say a good deal about the character and source of the change produced by TD therapy. Psychological studies by Hughes and Martin in combination with theoretical work by Michael and Bienvenue indicate the probability that TD therapy improves the functioning of the outer hair cells and/or their related neural structures. Physiological work by Hughes (1975) and Puharich and Lawrence (1969) has indicated at least two mechanisms wich might mediate that improved functioning--increased deep tissue blood flow and repolarization of cell membrane potentials. Finally, Bochenek and Bochenek have proven that TD therapy affects the VIII nerve action potential in a way consistent with the theory developed in this paper and long known to be related to hearing.

There is no longer any reason to doubt the efficacy of TD therapy. The empirical questions raised by early failures to replicate the original Puharich and Lawrence study have benn answered through careful methodological analysis of those papers and by further work. We now have experience with over 300 subjects (beyond those tested by Intellectron). Moreover, it is possible to give a rationale for the efficacy of the therapy which is grounded in a sophisticated and well-supported conception of sensorineural loss, and in physiological work involving TD therapy.

We know (Hughes) that 50% of persons with sensorineural hearing loss who are given TD therapy will show maintainable gains of 14% or more on PB word lists. We also know (Martin) that the before-after differences between percentages correct are even greater (30% to 40%) when the test used is more analogous to "real-life" situations (se Tables 1 a 2). We know, moreover, that these gains will be the most apparent in situations where there is background noise or where the to-be-perceived stimulus is close to threshold intensity. Finally, we know that it is in just these situations that persons with sensorineural hearing loss have traditionally reported the most difficulty. It appears, therefore, that the TD therapy holds significant promise for the treatment of sensorineural hearing disorders.

References

Bochenek, Z., and Bochenek, W., Electrocochleographic findings in patients with sensorineural hearing loss treated by transdermal electrostimulation. Presented at International Congress on Audiology, Florence, Italy (October 1976).

Brooks, S. and Harrison, R., An investigation of the efficacy of transdermal therapy on sensorineural hypacusis. Tranactions of AAOO (1974).

DeBoer, E., Measurement of the critical bandwidth in cases of perception deafness. Proc. III Int. Cong. Acoust. I: 100 (1961).

Eckberg, T., The application of the otostim procedure using the TD instrument for the restoration of sensorineural impairment. Presented at AAOO convention in Dallas, Tex. (1972).

Gerkin, G.M., Glorig, A. and Roeser, R.J., Transdermal electrostimulation therapy. Archives of Otolaryngol. 100: 96-99 (1974).

Glattke, T.J. and Simmons, F.B., Transdermal therapy and monosyllabic word discrimination. Archives of Otolaryngol. 100: 91-95 (1974).

Hughes, E.C., Arthur, R.A. and Whitaker, C.W., Electrostimulation for sensorineural hearing impairment: subject characteristics and protocol variations. Presented at Neuroelectric Society Meeting, New Orleans (1974)

Hughes, E.C., Arthur, R.H. and Whitaker, C.W., Transdermal electrostimulation and sensory hearing loss. Archives of Otolaryngol. 100: 100-106 (1974).

Hughes, E.C., Effect of TD electrostimulation and sensorineural loss in the "mild-moderate" ranges (i.e., less than 55dB). Unpublished report, January 1975. Also, Hughes, E.C., Effect of modulated electrostimulation on blood flow to tissues. Unpublished report, February 1975

Jerger, J. and Thelin, J.Bull. of Prosthetic Res. Pp.159-197 (Fall 1968).

Jerger, J., Burney and Crump. Predicting hearing loss from the acoustic reflex. J Spch. Area Disorders. 39: 11(1974)

Kohut, A., The effects of transdermal therapy on the perception of masked pure tones by sensorineural patients. A Master's Paper, Dept. of Speech Path. and Audio. P.S.U. (1976)

Martin, J.E. et al. Electrostimulation and sensorineural hearing loss: a preliminary report. J. Comm. Dis. 6: 145-150 (1973).

Michael, P.L. and Bienvenue, G.R., A procedure for early detection of noise-susceptive individuals. Amer. Industrial Hygiene Assoc. Jour. Pp. 55-55 (January 1976).

Nelson, D.G., An evaluation of the synthetic syntax sentence test. Thesis, Vanderbilt University (1968).

Paparella, M. and Melnik, W. Stimulation deafness. P. 427 in Sensori-Neural Hearing Processes and Disorders. A. Graham (Ed.), Little-Brown Company, Boston (1967).

Prout, J.H., Electrostimulation as a therapy for sensorineural hearing loss. Presented at Amer. Acoustical Society Convention (1976).

Puharich, H.K. and Lawrence, J.L., Hearing rehabilitation by means of transdermal electrotherapy on human hearing loss of sensori-neural origin. Acta Otolaryngol. 67: 69-83 (1969). See also, Reed, G.E., Puharich, H.K., Cortes, L.E., Brewster, W.R. and Lawrence, J.L. Electrodynamic approach to thrombus prevention in a ventricular assist device. Circulation 38, Suppl.6: 162 (1968).

Rosenthal, R. Experimenter Effects in Behavioral Research. New York: Appleton-Century-Crofts (1966).

Scharf, B. and Hellman, R. A model of loudness summation Applied to impaired ears. J. Acoust. Soc. Amer. 40: 71 (1966).

Spoendlin, H. Innervation of the cochlear receptor. Pp. 185 in Basic Mechanisms of Hearing A.R. Moller (Ed.), Academic Press, New York (1973).

Tonndorf, J. Transdermal electrostimulation therapy. Archives of Otolaryngol.100: 107-108 (1974).

Von Bekesy, G. Neural inhibition units of the eye and skin. Quantitative description of contrast phenomena. J.Opt. Soc. Amer. 50: 1060 (1960).

Von Bekesy, G. Experiments in Hearing. P. 207. McGraw-Hill, New York (1960b).

Von Bekesy, G. Lateral inhibitions of heat sensations on the skin. J. Applied Physiol. 17: 1003 (1962).

Chapter 4

Real-Ear Measures of Hearing Aid Performance

Geary A. McCandless, Ph.D.

In 1975 Harris reported "...there is no ready way to specify the real-ear frequency response characteristics of an aid. The manufacturer's data on the aid are from a 2-cc coupler, not a true artificial ear, and the differences between coupler data and the condition of the patient's eardrum are known to be significant and even to render the manufacturer's data misleading". While it is true the 2-cc coupler was intended to simulate the acoustic characteristics of the average ear wearing a hearing aid, it is well known that few ears are "average", making the assumptions of the 2-cc coupler rather tenuous in many instances. In terms of physical volume, general configuration, and diameter, ears vary considerably. Also, in considering the total sound spectra which reaches the eardrum, many other intervening factors must be countered as influences on the auditory spectra reaching the ear via a hearing aid, body baffle, canal resonance, microphone position (Berland and Nielson, 1969), type of earmold, depth of mold, and length of the sound tube (Lybarger, 1967).

Despite the inherent problems associated with couplers, it should not be inferred that they are valueless. In many instances the 2-cc coupler response is very close to that measured in the ear canal (Martin, 1971). More importantly it provides a standard measurement by which manufacturers and researchers can compare and express in a uniform way frequency response curves and other measures. Its major limitation is that the 2-cc coupler initiates a closed-mold system and cannot adequately quantify hearing aid performance with open or vented ear molds or sound tubes in the ear canal.

In order to really understand the ultimate effects on speech discrimination, loudness comfort, subjective quality and perhaps other factors, it seems obvious that the performance of a hearing aid must be measured as it is influenced by the source of a sound, the characteristics of the environment, acoustic properties of the external ear and canal, as well as all the "plumbing" attached to the aid. This implies the best way to objectively quantify the total amplification and acoustic system is to make measurements at the eardrum.

The use of manikins such as Kemar (Burkhard, 1976), which simulate the average head and ear is an interim step to real-ear measures, but as with the 2-cc coupler, it also represents an "average" ear. Too many clinical patients deviate sufficiently from the manikin norms to make precise inferences of gain, frequency response or saturation sound pressure level (SSPL). The Kemar concept has real value, however, for studying many hearing aid parameters such as open molds, venting and effects of sound location, and acoustic environment. Further, it has the advantage that free-field tests are stable and reproducible, is easily calibrated, and shows no fatigue.

Real-ear measures using probe microphone coupler versus real-ear measures were reported as early as 1944 (LeBel, 1944). Luter Ewartson (1957) reported real-ear measures using a probe microphone to be very similar to those in the 2-cc coupler. Still later, Sacks and Burkhard (1972), Bryant (1972) and others have found differences of 3-15 dB between probe microphone and coupler valves primarily at frequencies above 2000Hz. These differences were felt to be of sufficient magnitude to influence hearing aid function and subjective quality judgements.

The use of real-ear measures with probe microphones has been particularly useful in identifying effects of no-mold or open mold fittings. The probe microphone technique, for example, has helped identify subtle enhancement of high frequencies due to properties of the pinna and ear canal (Djupesland and Zwislocki, 1977) and effects of ear canal diameter and insert tip size (Courtois and Berland, 1972). The probe microphone technique has the disadvantage of requiring specially prepared earmolds and immobilization of the subject in order that the small probe tube can be properly inserted and maintained at a constant position in the ear canal. As presently used, this technique is obviously inappropriate for general clinical use, especially on active children or others who are unable to remain motionless during the test.

Attempts to overcome the technical problems associated with probe measurements have been made by using small electret microphones inserted between the earmold and ear drum (Vernon, 1978). The small size of the external canal also makes this procedure impractical for children. In many instances the insertion of the microphone is tactically difficult and sometimes requires an operating microscope for proper placement.

There is little doubt that the real-ear measures described above have added immeasurably to our knowledge of the combined effects of certain acoustic and electroacoustic systems. Much yet remains to be learned regarding these interactions. Most needed is a technique which takes relatively little time to perform and which can be used as a final check on the acoustic signals reaching the eardrum. Only at that time will clinicians be able to relate electroacoustic properties to subjective estimates of sound quality and hearing aid use.

Real-Ear Measures Using Behavioral Responses From Aided and Unaided Thresholds

Ideally the real-ear gain at the eardrum should be measured on each potential candidate for amplification. The combination of hearing test results plus the physical measures in the ear canal would add the needed precision to the fitting process now lacking. More importantly, effects of earmolds, tubing, venting, or filters, etc. could be quantified. Unfortunately, probe or other microphone insertion techniques are not yet clinically practical. However, behavioral or electrophysiological responses from the subject can be utilized to determine gain, frequency response, and perhaps other characteristics of a hearing aid.

The earliest reported technique of determining real-ear data from behavioral responses was between 1942-45. Sound field audiometry was employed as a part of hearing aid evaluation procedures in several army hospitals to determine the use-gain of a hearing aid. Aided speech tests largely replaced free-field tests of hearing aid gain for many years, primarily because of fears of effects of standing waves and other difficulties in controlling and calibrating the pure tone stimuli. In 1958 Ross presented substantive evidence that pure tone thresholds obtained in free-field were valid and reliable especially if warble tones are used as stimuli. Further, Ross strongly recommended the use of free-field audiometry to measure the frequency response and gain of hearing aids while being worn by the subject.

Behavioral real-ear measures are determined simply by presenting warble tones or other stimuli free-field through a loudspeaker located in a sound attenuator room. Calibration can be done using a sound level meter with the microphone focused at the ear canal of a subject sitting in the test position, or clinical calibration can be derived from the average free-field thresholds for normal subjects (Duffy, 1978).

Figure 1 illustrates how real-ear gain and frequency response can be obtained by using the shift in the unaided versus the aided thresholds to free-field warble tone stimuli. The results are shown on a sound pressure chart. The results shown here are taken from a subject with a sloping high frequency hearing loss averaging 30 dB. With the hearing aid gain set at a comfort level, there is about 15 dB average gain for frequencies 500, 1000, and 2000 Hz at this volume level.

The chart at the right side of Figure 1 illustrates behavioral or free-field measured frequency response. The zero line is a reference level based on the unaided thresholds. The subject's hearing aid has about 5 dB per octave rise from 500-1000 and 10dB/octave from 1000 to 3000 Hz. This technique indicates the basic real-ear frequency response characteristics of the aid as well as the average gain at a comfort level setting. A family of frequency response curves can be derived by changing the volume control.

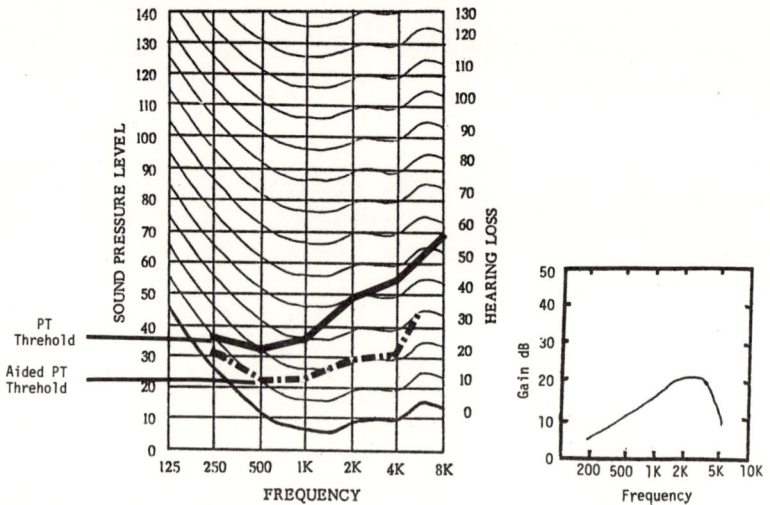

Figure 1. Real-ear gain as measured using the shift in unaided and aided free field thresholds. Also shown at right is the real-ear frequency response. The zero baseline or reference is the free field unaided pure tone threshold level.

Figure 2 shows the real-ear and 2-cc coupler response curves for this same hearing aid. The real-ear response clearly has less gain from about 1200-3000 Hz, the maximum difference being 8 dB at 1500 Hz. As might be expected, there tends to be a closer correspondence of functional gain to probe microphone measures than to those of functional gain to 2-cc coupler values. Still, slight differences between probe (insertion gain) and functional gain values have been reported by Preves and Orton (1978). They found that the two techniques always yielded gain values ± 5 dB for frequencies 250-6000 Hz. However, insertion gain was found to be slightly greater than functional gain at all frequencies, the mean difference ranging from .3 dB at 250 Hz and 6000 Hz to 4.6 dB at 5 KHz. The functional difference would appear to be due to impedance of the conducting system and psychophysiological transmission loss, or it may be due in part to the measurement techniques used. The concurrence between physically and biologically measured gain is really very encouraging since it tends to validate the behavioral derived real-ear gain technique.

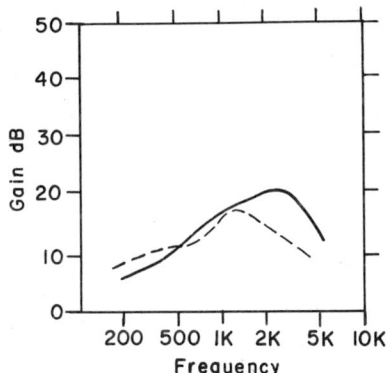

Figure 2. Real-ear and 2-cc coupler response curve for one hearing aid.

Since real-ear performance is based on subjective threshold tests, this technique is not really appropriate for measuring SSPL; however, subjective and loudness discomfort thresholds are appropriate measures of the upper functional intensity limit to which the SSPL in a hearing aid should correspond. Also the shift from the unaided to the aided level of loudness discomfort threshold (LDL) is still another measure of real-ear gain. Figure 3 illustrates how shifts in LDL thresholds yield both gain and frequency response data.

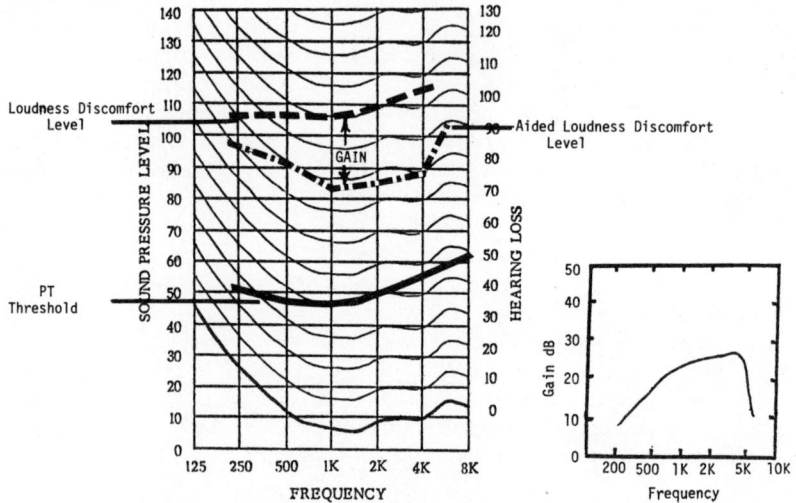

Figure 3. Illustration of how real-ear gain and frequency response data can be derived from loudness discomfort thresholds measured free field in the aided and unaided condition.

To summarize, the use difference scores for speech in an unaided vs. aided condition has long been used as an indication of gain for speech. Free field pure tone stimuli work equally well and have the added advantage of providing functional frequency response curves. Unaided-aided pure tone (or other stimuli) threshold information coupled with unaided-aided discomfort threshold, not only reflect functional gain, but also indicates the size of the patient's dynamic range as well as the effects of amplification on this range.

Real-Ear Performance Using Acoustic Reflex Measures

A more recent attempt to measure real-ear gain was reported by McCandless and Miller (1972), Tonnison (1975), and Snow and McCandless (1976) based on the shifts between the aided and unaided acoustic reflex (AR) thresholds in sound field. This technique can be used clinically to set the hearing aid volume for noncooperative subjects or to measure real-ear or functional gain and frequency response characteristics.

With this procedure pure tones, damped wave trains,

speech or other stimuli are presented free field via a loudspeaker. A probe from an electroacoustic impedance device is placed in the ear contralateral to the one wearing the aid as illustrated in Figure 4. Both aided and unaided reflex thresholds are measured as indicated on the compliance meter or read out on a recorder. Figure 5 shows the free field pure tone and acoustic reflex thresholds as well as the aided AR thresholds for a five year old child with a high frequency sensorineural hearing loss. Greater shifts in the reflex thresholds for the high frequencies suggested greater intensity compensation where the hearing loss is greatest. The chart at the right side of Figure 5 shows the real-ear gain using the unaided reflex thresholds as the zero reference level.

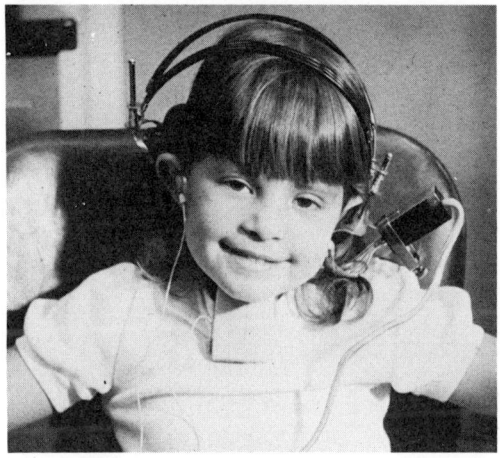

Figure 4. Photograph of aided reflex measures being taken on a five year old child. Note the impedance probe is placed in the ear contralateral to the hearing aid.

Figure 6 shows the free field pure tone and unaided and aided reflex thresholds for a 46 year old subject. The subject complained repeatedly that his aid sounded distorted and that speech was not clear. Measures using a 2-cc coupler failed to reveal any unusual electroacoustic characteristics. The frequency response is shown at right in Figure 6. Gain measures using the reflex technique revealed a significant dip centered at 1000 Hz which disappeared using a stock earmold. The mold and tubing were modified and the tests repeated, the results of which are also on Figure 6. The 1000 Hz dip was reduced and subjectively the aid was very accepta-

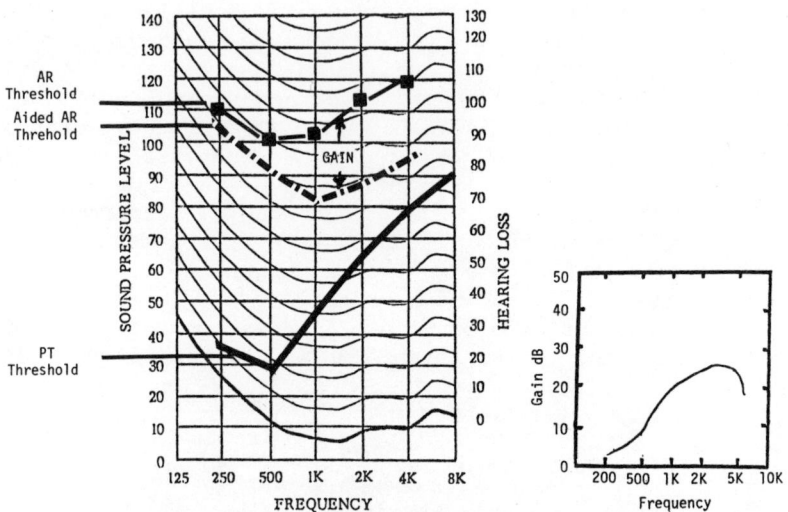

Figure 5. Free field pure tone and acoustic reflex thresholds from a 5 year old child with a high frequency sensorineural loss. The amount of shift in the AR threshold from the unaided to the aided condition indicates the amount of real-ear gain for this hearing aid.

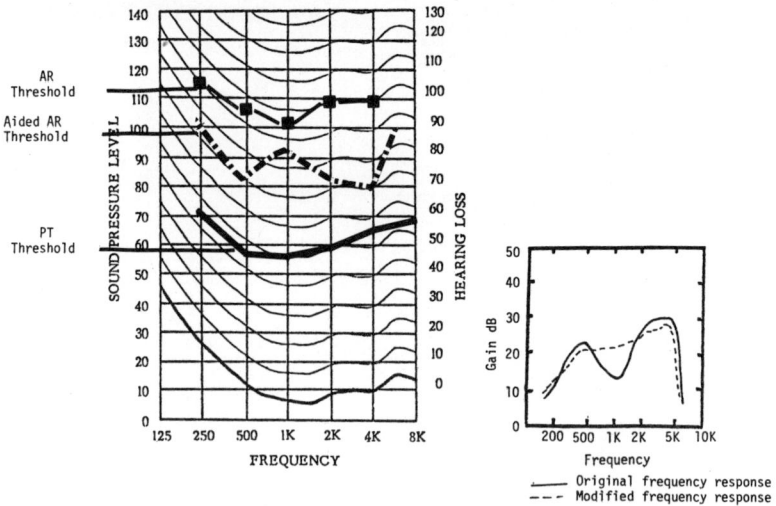

Figure 6. The free field pure tone and unaided and aided reflex thresholds are shown in SPL. Note the reduced gain at 1000 Hz compared with adjacent frequencies.

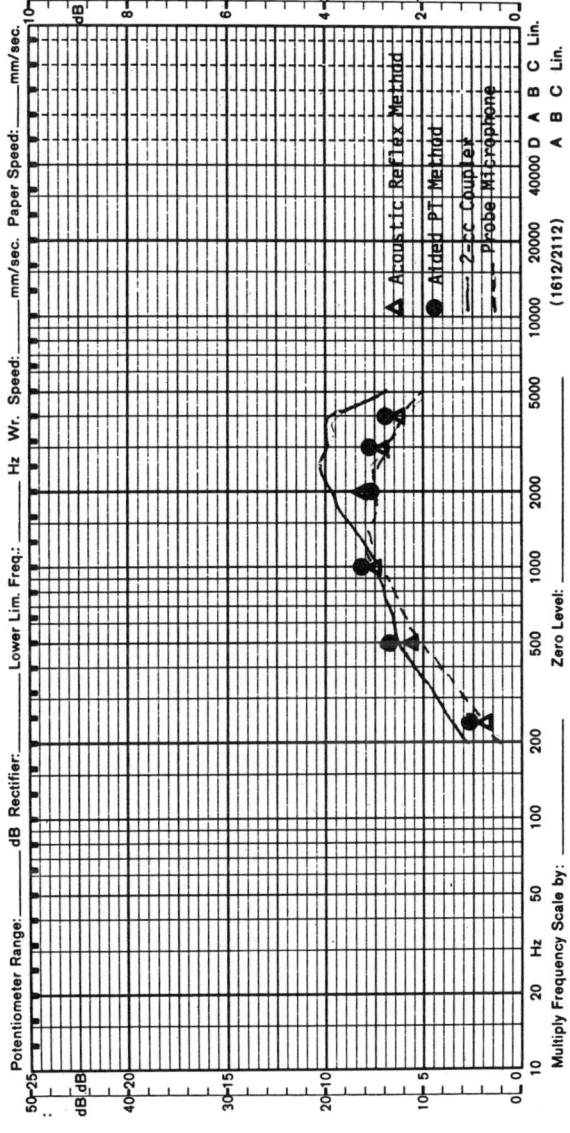

Figure 7. Comparison of the gain and response curve using four measurement techniques; probe microphone, 2-cc coupler, aided pure tone thresholds and aided acoustic reflex thresholds.

ble.

Tonisson (1975) indicated about a 5 dB enhancement in the gain at about 1000 Hz. This agrees well with our findings except that in our laboratory we find real-ear gain to be 2-4 dB higher than 2-cc coupler or probe microphone measures for frequencies up to 3000 Hz. Our data agree well with Preves and Orton (1978) in this respect.

Figure 7 is a typical comparison of the gain for one subject as measured by four techniques: 2-cc coupler, probe microphone, aided-unaided pure tone thresholds and acoustic reflex methods. While differences do occur, none were greater than 5.6 dB in this subject.

Other Applications of Real-Ear Measures

Speech stimuli can also be used to calculate gain, using either free field aided and unaided differences or using the acoustic reflex technique. Rainville (1977), Snow and McCandless (1976) and Keith (1978) use the speech AR to set gain by presenting speech at 60 dB SPL free field, then increasing the hearing aid volume until the reflex is just observed. Tato and Rainville (1976) also set the aid on full volume, then gradually increase the speech stimulus in sound field until the AR is seen. This yields a type of maximum gain value and can also be used with pure tones, narrow-band, and other stimuli.

Differential testing of gain and frequency response is easily accomplished using free field aided and unaided thresholds and acoustic reflex measures. Figure 8 demonstrates the difference in real-ear gain and frequency response for two different hearing aids. Aid B is seen to have greater gain, especially at 2000 Hz than Aid A.

Real-ear measures can be used for special applications which may have more research than clinical value. For example, a family of real-ear AR curves can be derived by increasing the volume control in 5 dB steps. In this way saturation and compression characteristics can be observed or influenced by the auditory system.

Summary

Four methods of real-ear measure have been reviewed: (1) probe microphone, (2) intra canal microphone placement, (3) unaided-aided free field thresholds, and (4) unaided and aided acoustic reflex thresholds. Individual variances are seen among these various techniques; however, they show fair-

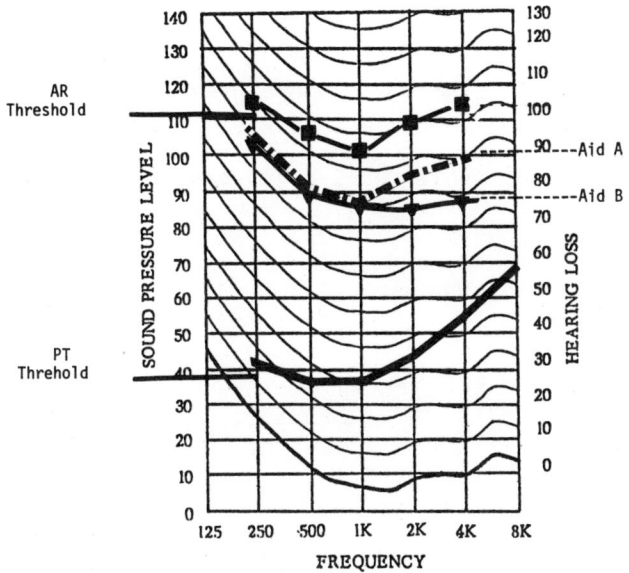

Figure 8. Difference in gain and frequency configuration using the AR technique for two hearing aids tested on the same subject. Note Aid B to have greater gain than Aid A especially at 2000 Hz.

ly good agreement, the deviations usually being less than 5 dB. They all show better inter-test agreement than with 2-cc coupler measures. This is to be expected since they reflect the acoustic characteristics of the pinna, ear canal, ear mold, head shadow, etc. and the coupler, one that does not.

When used as a clinical tool, behavioral or AR real-ear measures are well suited to reflect subtle effects of the electroacoustic and acoustic properties of the hearing aid system. These measures can be performed in a matter of a few minutes, and show excellent reliability. Being non-linguistic, they may have greatest value for children or non-cooperative subjects, and the AR measures can actually be obtained with a subject under sedation. These real-ear measures should not be limited to use with children, however, since they can be of great value in verifying effects of fine electroacoustic adjustments of the hearing aid.

The equipment for functional and AR real-ear measures are found in most clinics today; therefore, special, rather expensive instruments are not required. There have been sufficient reports of successful use of these tests as to encourage wider clinical application as well as carefully controlled experimentation necessary for final validation.

References

Bereland, O. and Nielson, E., Sound pressure generated in the human external ear by a free field sound. Audecibel, 103-109 (1969).

Bryant, H.W., Comparable coupler and real ear measurements on supra-aural and insert type earphones., J. Acoust. Soc. Amer., 52, 1599-1606 (1972).

Burkhard, M.D., Kemar, a tool for hearing aid evaluation. Audecibel, 126-134 (1976).

Courtois, J. and Berland, O., No-mold fittings. Audecibel, 171-181- (1972).

Djupesland, G. and Zwislocki, J.J., Sound pressure distribution in the outer ear. Scandinavian Audiol. 1: No. 4 197-203 (1972).

Duffy, J.K. Sound field audiometry and hearing aid evaluation. Hearing Instruments, 6-12 (1978).

Harris, J.D., Hearing aid prescription - fact or fantasy. Hearing Instruments. Feb 11--12 (1975).

Keith, R.W., Sininger, L. New ideas in hearing aid selection. Hearing Instruments. 29, 6, 6-8/34 (1978).

LeBel, C.J. Pressure and field response of the ear in hearing aid performance determination. J. Acous. Soc. Am., 16: 63-67 (1944).

Lybarger, S., Ear-mold acoustics. Audecibel,9-19 (1967).

Martin, M.C., Are frequency characteristics important? Scandinavian Audiology, Suppl. 1 93-108 (1971).

McCandless, G.A. and Miller, D., Loudness discomfort and hearing aids. National Hearing Aid Journal. June 7-28-32 (1972).

Preves, D.A. and Orton, J.F., Use of acoustic impedance measures in hearing aid fitting. Hearing Instruments. June, 22-34 (1978).

Rainville, M., Hearing aid fittings using stapedial reflex measurements. Proc. of III International Symposium on Impedance Audiometry. Acton, Mass., American Electromedics Corp. 49-50 (1976).

Ross, M., Aided sound field audiograms. In M.C. Pollack (ed.) Amplification for the hearing impaired. N.Y., Grune and Stratton, 219-233 (1977).

Sachs, R.M. and Burkhard, M.D., Earphone pressure response in ears and couplers. Presented at the 83rd meeting of the Acoustical Society of America. Buffalo, N.Y. (1972).

Snow, T. and McCandless, G.A., The use of impedance measures in hearing aid selection. National Hearing Aid J.7/32-33 (1976).

Tato, J.M., Rainville, M.J., Utilization du reflexe stapedien pour l'adaptation des prostheses. <u>Audiology</u>. 15, 428-432 (1976).

Tonisson, W., Measuring in-the-ear gain of hearing aids by the acoustic reflex method. <u>J. Spch and Hrng. Res.</u> 18, 5-16 (1975).

Vernon, J., In-the-ear measures using an electret microphone. Presented at the Medical Audiology Otology Workshop, Vail, Colorado, March 1978.

Chapter 5

The Non-Universal Binaural Hearing Advantage

Bruce Siegenthaler, Ph.D.

Hearing with two ears generally is conceded to be better than hearing with one ear. For normals a 2.5 dB to 3.0 dB binaural advantage for speech reception and pure tone thresholds has been carefully documented, especially under earphones and when stimuli to the two ears are equated for sensation level (Keys, 1947; Shaw, Newman and Hirsh, 1947; Breakey and Davis, 1949).

Speech intelligibility also seems to be better with binaural than with monaural hearing. Norlund and Fritzell (1963) demonstrated this when the speech signal had very low information content and was almost unintelligible monaurally. Chappell, Kavanagh, and Zerlin (1963) found binaural speech intelligibility for normals to be better by twenty percent in an environment of conversation-like noise. Gelfand and Hochberg (1976) found better binaural speech intelligibility for normals and for hearing impaired subjects with symmetrical sensorineural hearing losses. The binaural advantage was larger for the normal group.

However, binaural listening does not necessarily show improvement over monaural listening when one or both ears are defective. Groen and Hellema (1962) found that while subjects with central deafness and subjects with normal hearing had binaural articulation curve slopes the same as their monaural articulation curve slopes, persons with peripheral deafness showed steeper articulation test curves for binaural than for monaural hearing. Further, Groen and Hellema (1963) reported that while among groups of subjects binaural listening resulted in average increase in articulation score and dynamic range, eighteen percent of the subjects with perceptive defects (sic) were better served by monaural than by binaural hearing.

Harris (1965) found that the improvement in intelligibility by dichotic rather than monotic mode of listening was 25 to 33 percent, but he also found that hearing via a defective ear and a normal ear in the stereophonic mode caused decrease in inteligility in comparison to hearing via the normal ear only. Dirks and Wilson (1969) found that while sensorineural loss and normal hearing persons can achieve better binaural than monaural hearing for speech in noise, the improvement is dependent upon the azimuths of the signal and of the noise being different. The binaural advantage is lost when both signal and noise come from the same source. Arkebauer, Mencher and McCall (1971), utilizing persons with hearing loss, found that for eight of their ten subjects speech discrimination was poorer binaurally than monaurally. When the poorer of the two ears of these subjects was occluded there was an increase in intelligibility. They observed a trend toward binaural speech intelligibility being better when the two ears were different than when the two ears were more alike in threshold.

Thus it appears that although among groups of listeners there is a mean improvement in hearing test score with binaural hearing, it is not so for all listeners nor under all listening conditions.

Boca, Teatini and Antonelli (1964), and Hayashi, Ohta and Morimato (1966) described binaural fusion as essential to the binaural hearing advantage. Acoustic signals are first processed separately at the peripheral ears, and later cross-analyzed, fused or integrated at a cortical or sub-cortical level. Arkebauer, Mencher and McCall (1971) speculated that because hearing loss causes distortion in signal processing by the peripheral ears, distorted signals are delivered to the central nervous system. When the CNS is required to handle two distorted inputs a too high demand for integration is placed on the system, and intelligibility suffers. Occluding one ear reduces the CNS integration problem and may result in improved intelligibility score.

In view of the several exceptions to the rule that binaural is equal to or better than monaural hearing, it is appropriate to look again at whether two-ear hearing is better than one-ear hearing, especially as the testing is done in audiology clinics. Drawing subjects from ongoing audiology clinical programs has the merit of providing a field test of the hypothesis that two-ear hearing is better than one-ear hearing as it applies to the auditory habilitation or rehabilitation of hearing impaired people, the population which is the raison d'etre of most audiology clinics.

Procedure

Data were obtained from two sources: consecutive case records of The Pennsylvania State University Speech and Hearing Clinic, and consecutive reports from audiology clinics cooperating with a state-wide agency which has a hearing aid procurement program in Pennsylvania. The data were SRT and speech intelligibility maximum scores for each ear, and binaural SRT and intelligibility maximum scores. Complete sets of tests scores were not available on all subjects. The total sample was 179 subjects, all over 16 years of age. None was suspect of functional hearing loss, neurological disorders other than sensorineural hearing loss, or unusual hearing conditions. The binaural testing was either in a sound field or under earphones. Although the mixture of conditions under which the data were collected detracts from strict experimental control, they provide a sample of people as they are tested in the normal practice of audiology. Inspection of the raw test scores indicated no trend toward either earphone or sound field testing causing a bias in the data. The two sets of data provided (a) a well controlled condition, and (b) a general field-program condition.

Table 1 shows mean and range of SRT and speech intelligibility scores of the subjects. No interpretation should be made as to relationships between monaural and binaural test scores in Table 1 because the means are across all subjects and are not sensitive to differences among nor within subjects.

Table 1. Mean and range of hearing test scores.

	Penn State		Agency	
	Mean	Range	Mean	Range
SRT in dB re Normal				
	(N97)		(N82)	
Right	42.3	-5 to 105	58.6	20 to 105
Left	38.5	-5 to 100	58.4	5 to 100
Binaural	30.6	0 to 80	51.1	5 to 100
Maximum Intelligibility in % Correct				
	(N66)		(N44)	
Right	77.6	0 to 96	74.7	12 to 96
Left	78.6	0 to 98	62.1	4 to 96
Binaural	82.4	32 to 98	71.5	16 to 100

Table 2. Number, percent, and mean difference between binaural and better ear SRT scores.

db Differences Between Binaural and Better Ear		Penn State			Agency			All Subjects	
	N	% of Total N	Mean dB Diff.	N	% of Total N	Mean dB Diff.	N	% of Total N	Mean dB Diff.
Binaural worse than Better Ear	5	10	10.3	5.0	3	6.1	4.4	13	8.4	4.8
	4	0			1			1		
	3	0			1			1		
Binaural same as Better Ear	2	0	50.5		2	78.0		2	63.1	
	0	49			54			103		
	2	0			8			8		
Binaural better than Better Ear	4	0	39.2	5.5	4	15.8	5.8	4	28.5	5.6
	5	34			6			40		
	10	4			3			7		
Total N		97			82			179		

Table 3. Number, percent, and mean difference between binaural and better ear maximum intelligibility scores.

% Intelligibility Difference between Binaural and Better Ear	Penn State			Agency			All Subjects	
	N	% of Total N	Mean % Diff.	N	% of Total N	Mean % Diff.	% of Total N	Mean % Diff.
Binaural worse than Better Ear								
44	0			1	11.4	23.2	4.5	23.2
28	0			1				
20	0			1				
12	0			2				
Binaural same as Better Ear								
8	10			3				
6	13			0				
4	15			4				
2	8			5				
0	4	100		13	86.4		94.6	
2	6			8				
4	4			5				
6	2			0				
8	4			0				
Binaural better than Better Ear								
16	0			1	2.3	16.0	.9	16.0
Total N	66			44			110	

93

The difference in SRT between binaural and better of the two ears, and the difference in maximum intelligibility between binaural and better of the two ears were calculated for each subject. Tables 2 and 3 show the difference-score distributions.

Analysis

Two dB was taken as the error of estimate for SRT scores, and 8 percent was taken as the error of estimate for intelligibility scores. Only differences between test scores greater than these values were considered to be reliable.

A majority of the cases had monaural and binaural test score differences within errors of estimate, but the following important exceptions occurred:

1. In the Penn State data 49.5 percent of the subjects had a difference greater than 2 dB between the binaural and the better ear SRT; 10.3 percent had worse binaural than monaural SRT, and 39.2 percent had better binaural than monaural SRT.

2. In the Agency data 22 percent of the subjects had an SRT difference greater than 2 dB; 6.1 percent had worse binaural than monaural test scores, and 15.8 percent had better binaural than monaural SRT.

3. Among all subjects 36.1 percent had greater than 2 dB difference between binaural and better ear threshold; 8.4 percent had worse binaural than monaural test scores, and 28.5 percent had better binaural than monaural SRT.

4. In the Penn State data no subject had a difference between binaural and better ear intelligibility greater than 8 percent.

5. In the Agency data 13.7 percent of the subjects had a difference greater than 8 percent between binaural and better ear maximum intelligibility; 11.4 percent had worse binaural than monaural intelligibility test scores, and 2.3 percent had better binaural than monaural speech intelligibility.

6. Among all subjects 5.4 percent had a difference more than 8 percent in maximum intelligibility between better ear and binaural test scores; 5.4 percent had worse binaural than

than monaural speech intelligibility, and .9 percent had better binaural than monaural speech intelligibility.

To test for relationships among difference scores and several test scores product moment correlations were computed:

r between (difference between SRT of each subject's two ears) and (difference between better ear SRT and binaural SRT)

r between (difference between intelligibility of each subject's two ears) and (difference between better ear intelligibility and binaural intelligibility)

r between (better ear SRT) and (difference between better ear SRT and binaural SRT)

r between (better ear intelligibility) and (difference between better ear and binaural intelligibility)

r between (better ear SRT) and (difference between better ear and binaural intelligibility)

The range of r values was -.18 to .16. None was significant at the .05 level nor satisfactory as a predictor of difference between monaural and binaural test scores.

Conclusion

The data indicate that while most persons have essentially the same binaural test scores for SRT and for maximum speech intelligibility as they have for the better of the two ears, some have discrepancies greater than errors of test measurement between the better ear and the binaural hearing test scores. The discrepancies are not always in the direction of better binaural than monaural test scores.

In the present data approximately three times as many persons (28.5 percent) had better binaural SRT scores compared to better-ear SRT scores, than had worse binaural SRT scores

(8.4 percent). The situation is reversed for speech intelligibility: about five times as many persons (4.5 percent) have worse binaural than monaural better-ear speech intelligibility than have better binaural speech intelligibility (.9 percent).

The findings are consistent for subjects with worse binaural than monaural test scores with the hypothesis that for some listeners when the two ears each feed a distorted signal into the central nervous system the auditory pathway is less able to handle the possibly conflicting information (produces poorer SRT and worse maximum intelligibility test scores) than when only one ear is functioning. That this should be more so for an intelligibility test than for a threshold test is likely in view of the greater redundancy in spondee words used for threshold tests, in contrast to the greater degree of difficulty and lesser redundancy of single-syllable intelligibility test words.

For subjects with better binaural than monaural test scores, the hypothesis of binaural summation may be a valid explanation of the findings.

Judging from the present data, factors such as difference in test scores between the individual ears or level of test score for the better ear are not predictors of how the binaural test scores are related to hearing in the better ear.

These data indicate that clinical evaluations of hearing performance ought to incorporate hearing test scores for each ear individually as well as for binaural listening because the hearing test scores for the better ear is not a reliable predictor of the individual's binaural hearing ability as measured for clinical audiology practice. Monaural hearing test scores as well as binaural test scores should be obtained for adequate measurement of the individual audiology clinic patient's hearing performance. This recommendation is especially appropriate when considering a hearing aid because of the possibility of poorer hearing rehabilitation with a binaural rather than a monaural hearing aid fitting.

REFERENCES

Arkebauer, H., Mencher, G. and McCall, C., Modification of speech discrimination in patients with binaural asymmetrical hearing loss, J. Spch. Hrg. Dis., 36, 208-212 (1971).

Bocca, E., Teatini, G., and Antonelli, A., Binaural hearing: fusion vs. separation, Int. Audio., 3, 193-196 (1964).

Breakey, M. and Davis, H., Comparisons of thresholds for speech: word and sentence tests; receiver vs. field and monaural vs. binaural hearing. Laryngoscope, 59, 236-250 (1959).

Chappell, R., Kavanagh, J. and Zerlin, S., Monaural vs. binaural discrimination for normal listeners, J. Spch Hrg. Res., 6, 263-269 (1963).

Dirks, D. and Wilson, R., Binaural hearing of speech for aided and unaided conditions, J. Acoust. Soc. Amer., 12, 650-664 (1969).

Gelfand, S. and Hochberg, I., Binaural and monaural speech discrimination under reverberation, Audiology, 15, 172-184 (1976).

Groen, J. and Hellema, A., Binaural speech audiometry, Int. Audiol., 1, 218-221 (1962).

Groen, J. and Hellema, A., Binaural sprach-audiometry, Z. Horgorate-Akustik, 2, 160-165 (1963).

Harris, J., Monaural and binaural speech intelligibility and the stereophonic effect, Laryngoscope, 75, 428-444 (1965)

Hayashi, R., Ohta, F. and Morimato, M., Binaural fusion tests: a diagnostic approach to central auditory disorders, Int. Audiology, 5, 133-135 (1966).

Keys, J., Binaural vs. monaural hearing, J Acoust. Soc. Amer. 19, 629-631 (1947).

Norlund, B. and Fritzell, B., The advantages of binaural hearing for the understanding of speech, Acta Oto-laryng., Suppl. 188 (1963).

Shaw, W., Newman, E. and Hirsh, I., The difference between monaural and binaural thresholds, J. Exper. Psychol., 37, 229-242 (1947).

Chapter 6

The Otomandibular Syndrome

Ira M. Klemons, D.D.S.

There is renewed interest of late in what some refer to as "Holoistic Medicine". I say "renewed" because the concept of relating disease symptoms to seemingly unrelated pathosis in other body areas was key to the most ancient medical traditions. The ancient Ayurvedic school of India and the Chinese concepts of disease regarded first the unity of the body and then the diversity of its many parts. With this in mind the ancient physician did not find it strange, for example, to stimulate the foot to improve some malady of the head. Today, as more is being learned of the effects of stress, of nutrition and of nerve and muscle interrelationships, it is again becoming clear that symptoms of disease in different body areas may well have a single cause.

"Stress" as described by Selye is being implicated as a primary basis for an increasing number of disease processes. Selye demonstrated repeatedly that when an organism is subject to a demand, it responds by eliciting an "alarm reaction". This reaction, as you well know, includes a release of adrenalin and tensing of the muscles. In earlier societies this was often followed by a burst of action. A bear wandered into a cave and prehistoric man picked up a club, or ran the other way. In either case, the tension which developed was released through vigorous activity. Today this release is less likely to follow. Tensions develop at work, while commuting and at home, but most people remain sedentary. When you consider that the "alarm reaction" can be stimulated by an infinite variety of circumstances, be they physical, chemical or mental, many of the degenerative diseases currently prevalent can be seen in a new light. These pathological changes may be evident in any organ, and in any part of the body.

The development of symptoms varies in different individuals. A joint may be affected in one person first, while a gland is first affected in another. Adler and others have suggested that this variation is due to that organ being "inferior" in some respect. A genetic predisposition may make the kidney a weak link in the bodily system or an automobile accident may damage a shoulder, for example. Typically, under repeated stress, symptoms appear in this individual's "Target organ".

Certain organ systems seem to become targets especially frequently. It is estimated that 50% of all physician visits in the U.S. each year are for pains in the head. Gelb (1977) and others have found that as many as 80% of all head pains result from disorders of the muscles, ligaments and joints of the head and neck, especially the temporomandibular joints.

In fact, the vast majority of these head pains, upon closer observation appear to be associated with dysfunction in one or more other areas. Symptoms may include hearing loss, tinnitus, vertigo, stuffiness, pain or popping sounds in the ear.

According to Arlen (1977), these symptoms are normally unilateral. Patients usually find it difficult to localize the pain and describe it as "deep". Pain radiating to the sternocleidomastoid is typical. Sore throat, burning tongue, pressure in the eyes, irregular menstrual cycle, elevated blood pressure, forgetfulness and insomnia are also quite common.

This rather impressive list of seemingly unrelated symptoms often causes the unfortunate patient to seek specialist after specialist. Neurological, ENT, orthopedic, dental and psychiatric offices are familiar to many who suffer from this syndrome. Brain scans, tranquilizers, hearing aids, ergotamines, narcotics and psychotherapy are usually employed in diagnosis or treatment. Yet the organ most directly responsible is the dysfunctional temporomandibular joint. Evaluation must include the following:

1. Does the patient have an obvious dental problem such as missing teeth or loose dentures?

2. When opening and closing the mouth, does the mandible deviate to one side? Such deviations are due to spasms of the muscles of mastication.

3. How wide does the patient open? The distance between the upper and lower teeth should be at least 40mm in the normal individual.

4. Does the patient experience clicking or popping sounds in the joint when opening or closing?

5. Does the patient grind or grit the teeth during the day or night?

6. Place your fingers with the nails facing backwards into the ear canals bilaterally and ask the patient to open and close. Pain along the anterior wall is likely to be due to an inflamed joint capsule. The location of the condyle is especially important. You should not feel a significant narrowing of the ear canal when your patient closes. Figure 1 shows the location of the condylar head in relation to the

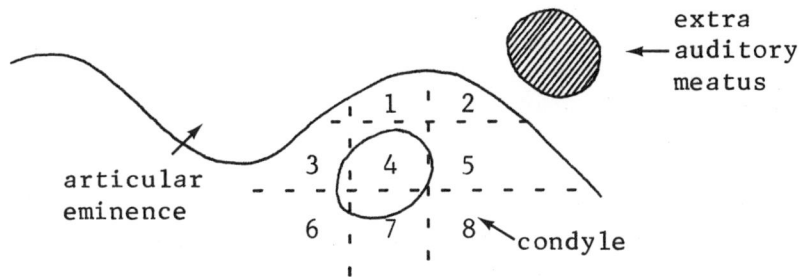

Figure 1. This condyle is pictured in the correct "4-7" position.

meatus and articular eminence. Gelb (1977) has devised a means of dividing the fossa to describe the location of the condyle. The position most likely to be symptom free overlaps squares 4 and 7. The condyle of the patient with otomandibular syndrome is displaced superiorly and posteriorly. Note the infringement on the ear canal which must necessarily result from malposed condyle in Figure 2. This patient, who often has a unilateral conductive hearing loss on this side may also find it uncomfortable to wear a hearing aid. Fortunately, orthopedic repositioning of the condyle and restoration of the muscles to their physiologic length will also result in an improvement in hearing.

Yanick (1979) and Arlen (1977) found that impedance measurements and routine audiological tests are valuable in differential diagnosis of this condition. As Yanick has explained it, "Patients affected by the syndrome generally exhibit type C tympanograms with negative pressure peaks commonly in the area of minus 300mm water pressure. Audiograms reveal a significant low tone ear-bone gap of 15 to 35 dB. In most cases, acoustic reflex thresholds are elicited only at

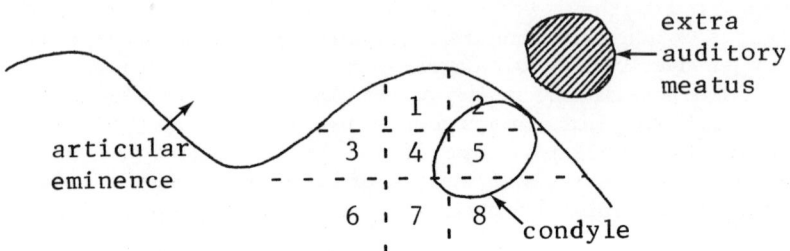

Figure 2. This condyle is pictured in a retruded and superior position, often associated with symptoms of the Otomandibular Syndrome.

the maximum compliance point or at the peak of the tympanogram. Static compliance values are generally below normal values".

It is interesting to note that in some cases pulsating spasms of the tensor tympani muscle can be observed by a deflecting needle on the impedance bridge.

Localizing our attention to the temporomandibular joint, let us review the anatomy. The condyle of the mandible is located within the Glenoid fossa and is separated from its bony roof above by the articular disc. The four major muscles of mastication (temporalis masseter, internal and external pterygoids) are close to this area. For these muscles to be at their physiologic lengths, the condyle must be in its correct position.

A variety of situations may prevent the condyle from returning to its rest position, however. Leaning against a hand while reading, cocking the head to hold the phone against a shoulder, or sleeping with the jaw forced to one side will all force the condyle out of its rest position. The loss of posterior teeth, incomplete eruption, and inappropriate treatment by orthodontists or other dentists, may predispose the individual to incorrect positioning of the jaw. Most commonly, tension and stress which is often released through grinding or gnashing of teeth, can be seen as responsible for this pathosis.

The loss of balance between the right side of the dental arch and the left side necessarily force the condyle of the affected side into a more retruded position. The muscles of mastication are no longer capable of maintaining their physiologic lengths. Under continued stress spasms develop. The vicious cycle of pain, spasm, dysfunction, pain spasm and further dysfunction has begun.

The ear canal, being so intimate with this joint, is affected by the inflammatory process which follows. Even more significant to the hearing specialist is the resulting effect on the tensor tympani muscle whose function is to tense the tympanic membrane by drawing it medially. This muscle develops embryonically from the same blastema as the internal pterygoid muscle. Both contract in response to the same nerve which branches from the mandibular branch of the trigeminal. The relationship between dysfunction in the ear and dysfunction of the TM joint result from the relationship between these two muscles. If the internal pterygoid goes into spasms, so will the tensor tympani. As a result impedance changes are observed with the tympanogram. According to Arlen (1977), these spasms may cause otalgia, a sense of fullness in the ear, tinnitis, hearing loss and disequilibrium.

A differential diagnosis must be made to determine the mode of treatment which is to be employed. Of course, otolaryngological disease must be ruled out initially. Assuming that the cause has been localized to the TM joint, it must be determined whether the patient is suffering from a true otomandibular syndrome or the myofascial pain dysfunction syndrome (MPD). In simple terms, it can be said that the MPD is acute while OMS is chronic. In MPD pain may at times be exquisite, no bony changes are noted on radiographs and the TMJ is not sensitive to palpation. If an MPD persists for over six months, and ear symptoms develop, it may be considered to be otomandibular syndrome.

Treatment of MPD may include massage of the muscles in spasm after spraying with ethyle chloride. Gentle exercises are helpful as well as correction of noxious habits and the use of a transcutaneous nerve stimulator such as the "Pain Suppressor". Adjustment of the bite to eliminate premature contacts as the mouth closes may also be useful.

The otomandibular syndrome requires additional treatment however. The patient suffering from OMS has lived with his or her condition for sometime. Frequently posterior teeth have been lost and the condyles have shifted into a non-physiologic position. Muscle spasm, trauma, and improper occlusion may cause the condyle to move into a superior or retruded position. This position, of course, is less physiologically healthy than the "4-7" position mentioned earlier. Compression of the articular disc results and osteoarthritis often develops.

Many generalized disturbances nay lead to this developing as a chronic degenerative process. Ask your patient whether her nails break easily, her skin is dry, whether she tires easily and whether she is particularly bothered by cold. If she answers "yes" to these questions she may well be hypothyroid. Blood tests may show the patient to be marginally normal but consultation with an endocrinologist is essential. Hypothyroidism, estrogen imbalance and other endocrine disturbances may contribute significantly to the seemingly localized muscle spasms which you are noting. In a situation such as this - which is not unusual - an endocrine disturbance can be said to be a contributing factor both to headaches and to the ear symptoms which otherwise might be thought to be unrelated.

Similarly, a diet high in refined carbohydrates and lacking essential vitamins and minerals, may contribute to the development of muscle spasms of the head and neck, especially when the mandible is malposed due to stress and poor occlusion.

The treatment of the otomandibular syndrome is based first and foremost on the orthopedic alignment of the jaws to each other. If we look at a human skull, we can bisect it in many different planes. For example, a mid-sagittal plane may be drawn through the face down its center. For correct balance, the mid-sagittal plane of the mandible must be continuous with the same plane of the maxilla. Similarly, four other planes may be established in an effort to analyze the face. Patients exhibiting symptoms of the otomandibular syndrome will be found not to have these planes of orientation in correct relation.

Patients suffering from otomandibukar syndrome must have these planes oriented through the use of orthopedic repositioning appliances for treatment to be successful in the long run. A myriad of treatment modalities may be attempted, but if the condyles of the mandible are not placed into their correct position and appropriate harmony brought to the related muscles and bones, the problem will often return. It may, however, seem in a different organ.

The orthopedic mandibular repositioning appliance is used to align the planes of orientation and cause the condyle to return to the "4-7" position when the mouth is closed. It is constructed after taking study models of the patient. The planes of orientation are drawn onto the casts and related on an articulator. The patient's true occlusion is of little concern because even if the occlusion is perfect by normal standards, the position of the jaw is incorrect. A wax impression of this new relationship is then made and transferred to the patients mouth. With it in position the condyles are no longer palpable through the ears. The appliance is then constructed of a cast chrome cobalt material and the occlusion surfaces are covered with acrylic. At the time the device is placed in the mouth it is balanced and adjustments are made to insure that the patient can chew properly. In many cases, the patient leaves the office symptom free. Because the appliance allows the masticatory muscles to achieve their physiologic length, many muscle spasms are relieved. In most cases, however, muscle spasms and contributing factors must be treated as well. The treatment modalities which follow, are also useful in treating the acute patient, the patient with myofascial pain dysfunction previously described who suffers from muscle spasms and associated radiating pain but has not as yet developed joint pathosis.

Muscles which remain in spasm may be treated in a variety of ways. Ethyl chloride spray, for example, may relieve pain and allow the patient to eliminate the spasm through gentle exercise. Muscles which have been in spasm for long periods of time may be scarred internally. They are referred to as "trigger points" and are successfully treated with injections of Lidocaine (without epinephrine) or with normal saline. Trigger points typically cause radiating or referred pain. The pressure of the fluid emanating from the hypodermic needle stimulates healing of the scarred tissue.

A variety of exercises may be used with great benefit. In conditions which have not yet degenerated to a chronic state, exercise alone is often adequate.

Clenching and grinding of the teeth place the organs of the mouth and its associated musculature under extraordinary stress. It is sometimes adequate for the health practitioner simply to recommend that the patient discontinue such habits. The following exercise may also be employed:

While sitting comfortably and timing yourself with a watch, close your mouth as tightly as possible for five seconds. Then relax every muscle in your body for five seconds. Repeat five times and practice three times per day. This exercise will help you develop an awareness of your jaw muscles. It will be easier to relax them whenever you notice that you are clenching during the day.

Relaxation of muscles in spasm may be achieved through the use of the following exercises:

1. While sitting comfortably, place your fist under your chin and try to open your jaw while exerting pressure against it. Hold in this position for five seconds, then relax all of your muscles for five seconds. Repeat five times and prac- three times per day.

2. While sitting comfortably place the tips of two fingers against the lower front teeth and pull downward. Simultaneously try to close your mouth. Hold for five seconds and then relax for five seconds. Repeat five times and practice three times per day.

Muscle spasms cause the jaw to shift to one side or the other when opening or closing. More harmonious functioning of the muscles will result from practice of the following exercise:

Break a toothpick in half and place the sharp end of one between the two front teeth of the upper jaw. Place the second toothpick between the two front teeth of the lower jaw. While watching in a mirror, open and close a maximum of one inch. Be sure to keep the lower toothpick moving in a straight, vertical line at all times. Practice for three minutes five times per day. Every two to three days open your mouth a little wider during the exercise.

Clicking of the joints when opening the mouth is due to an incorrect movement of the jaw. The TM joint should open like a hinge at first and then begin to slide forward. Many people habitually force the haw forward during its initial opening movement. This causes clicks and may cause pain. Show the patient the correct way to open and then have him practice the following exercises:

1. Hold your thumb against your upper front teeth and your index finger against your lower teeth while moving your fingers with a scissor-like motion. Stop if you experience pain. Repeat for three minutes, three times per day.

2. Curl your tongue upward and place the tip as far back as you can gainst the roof of your mouth. Open and close for three minutes while holding the tongue in this position. Practice three times per day.

Many people are uncertain of the correct position in which to close their jaws. In fact, the jaws should normally be apart. Over-awareness of occlusal relationships often predispose the patient to bruxing and should be discouraged. Throughout the day, the patient should think "lips together, teeth apart". In addition, while falling asleep she should suggest to herself, "If I grind my teeth, I will wake up". This positive statement is far more helpful than the negative suggestion, "I will not grind my teeth".

Two electronic instruments which are helpful in this treatment are the "Electrogalvanic Stimulator", and the "Pain Suppressor".

The Electrogalvanic Stimulator delivers high voltage pulses to the involved muscles over a range of frequencies. Tonic contraction or spasm is induced through proper use.

This can be used to tone the muscle and relieve pain.

The Pain Suppressor is a low voltage, high frequency instrument which interferes with the sensation of pain in the brain without the active response of the muscle.

A variety of techniques are available which aid the individual to relax and thus reduce the effects of stress. Biofeedback is quite helpful in aiding the individual to relax muscles or alter a variety of specific physiologic functions.

The Transcendental Meditation technique (TM) has a generalized effect on the body and mind. It is excellent as a preventive or therapeutic modality. The technique of TM is easily learned, does not require special equipment and can be practiced anywhere by anyone with a minimum of training. The TM technique has been studied extensively by biological and social scientists and has been found to aid the individual to use more of his potential in each of these areas. With respect to temporomandibular joint pathosis, improvement is thought to result from the increased ease with which practitioners of the Transcendental Meditation technique appear to deal with what were previously thought to be stressful situations. In addition, electromyograms and galvanic skin response are considerably lower after even a short period of practice.

The patient's nutritional state must not be overlooked. A diet high in refined carbohydrates or deficient in protein, vitamins or minerals predisposes the individual to many of the symptoms mentioned earlier. The patient's diet record should be evaluated by competent personnel trained in nutrition.

An endocrine disorder may also predispose the patient to Otomandibular Syndrome. If you are suspicious, especially of a hypothyroid or estrogen disturbance, referral to an endocrinologist is essential.

Habits mentioned earlier such as holding the telephone against the shoulder by tilting the head, or leaning against a hand while reading or watching TV place strain on the muscles of the face and neck. Sleeping on one's stomach may have the same effect. The patient should be counseled to eliminate such noxious habits.

Medication is rarely needed in the treatment of Otomandibular Syndrome although muscle relaxing drugs, narcotics and tranquilizers are often unnecessarily prescribed. The patient who insists on medication should be given two plain aspirin every four hours to reduce inflamation and pain.

Summary

The Otomandibular Syndrome is a frequently occurring disturbance of the ear which results from dysfunction of the temperomandibular joint and its associated musculature. Patients may experience hearing loss, tinnitis and fullness or pain in the ears which is often unilateral. Other symptoms may include pain, clicking or swelling of the TM joint, myospasm, headache, neck, shoulder or back pain, tingling or numbness of the arms, chronic sore throat, dizziness and burning sensations in the mouth. Treatment requires orthopedic repositioning of the mandible through the use of an intraoral appliance. Treatment of the musculature and generalized predisposing factors which may be endocrine or nutritional in origin must be considered. Techniques which help the individual to cope with the stress of daily life are of significant importance to overall success.

References

Arlen, H., The otomandibular syndrome, in Clinical Management of Head, Neck and TMJ Pain and Dysfunction, Gelb, H., Editor, Saunders Pub. Co., Phila., (1977).
Gelb, H., Clinical Management of Head, Neck and TMJ Pain and Dysfunction, Saunders Pub. Co., Phila., (1977).
Yanick, P., personal communication, Jan. 1979.

Chapter 7

Digital Processing Techniques in Speech Discrimination Testing
(Critical Band Measurements for Use in Hearing Aid Testing)

Gordon R. Bienvenue, Ph.D. and Paul L. Michael, Ph.D.

Recruitment and Critical Bands

The presence of non-linearities in the perception of loudness by patients with noise-induced hearing loss was first noted by Haberman (1890) in his now classic paper on "boilermaker's disease". The phenomenon was named recruitment by E.P. Fowler (1928) and was defined as an abnormally rapid increase in loudness (sound magnitude as perceived by a listener) when the sound level is increased. Stated otherwise, a given increase in sound level created a greater increment in the sensation of loudness for the recruiting ear than for the non-recruiting ear. A person with recruitment experiences extreme annoyance for loud sounds and a decreased range of sound levels that are comfortable for listening. Speech sounds are distorted and sound "foggy" or "blurred". Fowler (1963) characterized the most common difficulty of the recruiting listener: "The result is he will say, 'Do not shout at me', and yet if you lower your voice, even a trifle, he will say, 'Don't mumble', or 'I can't hear your voice, it seems loud enough, but I cannot understand what you are saying'."

Having defined the phenomenon of recruitment, Fowler went on to observe that it was absent in cases of middle ear pathology and concluded that the phenomenon arose from some neural malfunction of the hearing mechanism (1928, 1936, 1937, 1938). In 1948, Dix, Hallpike, and Hood were able to refine Fowler's conclusion by demonstrating that the recruitment phenomenon was limited to cases of cochlear end organ pathology. This finding has been supported by Luscher (1950), Eby and Williams (1951), and Dix (1965). Indeed, Harris (1953) noted that those pathologies showing loudness recruitment involve some mechanical damage within the cochlea as contrasted with a strictly neural dysfunction. Mygind (1950) shares this view suggesting that recruitment is indicative of a "conductive impairment" within the cochlea. Thus, it is generally agreed that the phenomenon of loudness recruitment is a pathological manifestation caused by structural injury to the cochlea.

The phenomenon of loudness recruitment appears paradoxical in that the ear with noise induced injury is in fact more sensitive to one parameter of sound than is the normal ear. This apparent contradiction may be reconciled by reference to critical bands. The critical band may be defined as some frequency band-width beyond which a listener's subjective response will change. In terms of loudness perception, the loudness sensation produced by random noise signals having bandwidths equal to or smaller than the critical band will appear to be constant if the sound pressure level of the noise is held constant. As the bandwidth is increased beyond that of the critical band, however, the perception of loudness increases even though the overall sound pressure level of the signal remains constant.

In contrast with the phenomena of recruitment and noise-induced hearing loss, current concepts on the morphological basis for critical bands and their disruptions remain speculative. Bekesy (1960, 1962) has suggested that the tuning of critical bands is too fine (i.e., bands are too narrow) to result solely from the vibrational characteristics (mechanical tuning) of inner ear structures. He proposes that the mechanical tuning within the inner ear is sharpened by a neural inhibition process. In such a model the region within the cochlea corresponding to one critical band is surrounded by a region where response to stimulation is inhibited. Obviously, such a neural inhibition model for frequency analysis at the cochlea would require a neural inhibitory mechanism. The presence of such a mechanism has long been recognized in the auditory system, but its specific function has never been clearly defined.

In 1942, Rasmussen drew attention to the efferent component of the auditory nerve and precisely traced the efferent fibers that innervate the cochlea. This pathway originates in the region of the superior-olivary nuclei of the brainstem and terminates within the cochlea. Consequently, it was named the olivo-cochlear bundle. In an overview of existing literature on olivo-cochlear feedback, Fex (1967) pointed out

that the primary function of the cochlear efferents seemed
to be inhibitory in nature. Thus, it is apparent that the
olivo-cochlear bundle of Rasmussen provides a cochlear inhibitory function and may be the mechanism for neural sharpening of critical bands posited by Bekesy. Before considering
this theory further, it will be useful to further examine
the innervation patterns of the cochlea.

Several studies have examined the behavioral performance
of animals in which the action of the olivo-cochlear bundle
was blocked. Dewson (1968) demonstrated that monkeys with a
transected olivo-cochlear bundle showed significant reduction
in their ability to discriminate human vowel sounds in a
background of noise. Following the olivo-cochlear bundle
transection, the animals required much higher signal-to-noise
ratios in order to achieve the same discrimination performance they had produced prior to surgery. Also in 1968, Capps
and Ades found that following surgical interruption of the
olivo-cochlear bundle in squirrel monkeys, all test animals
showed a marked deficiency in frequency discrimination performance. Trahiotis and Elliott (1970) found that sectioning
the olivo-cochlear bundle resulted in increased masking effect of broad band noise on the detection of pure tone signals. Finally, Pickles and Comis (1973) applied atropine
sulfate locally to the cochlear nuclei. The drug acted to
raise all auditory thresholds, but masked thresholds were
raised by a greater amount than unmasked thresholds. In the
latter study, the application of atropine sulfate may be expected to have affected afferent as well as efferent fibers.
This explains why absolute as well as noise masked thresholds
were altered. Since the noise masked thresholds were altered
to a greater extent, one may presume that these are affiliated with efferent as well as afferent functioning, wheras the
less affected, unmasked thresholds rely simply on afferent
processes.

The implication of the series of behavioral studies described above is the key to the critical bandwidth mechanism
proposed herein. Two observations were made in those studies
where efferent innervation to the cochlea was blocked;
    a) reduction in frequency discrimination ability, and
    b) reduction in the ability to recognize signals in a
       background of noise.
These two observations are closely related manifestations of
a single phenomenon. The recognition of a signal in a background of noise is dependent upon the frequency resolution
capabilities of the listener. The finer the resolution of the
ear (i.e., the narrower the passband of the ear as a filter)
the more noise the ear can reject. This means that only the

noise in a narrow frequency band centered around the signal serves to interfere with or mask its perception. The narrower the filtering, the less noise produces masking and, consequently, the lower the signal-to-noise ratio which can be tolerated. Conversely, any action which reduces the ability to recognize signals in noise or which requires higher signal-to-noise ratios for performance of the recognition task may be characterized as an action which reduces the resolution capabilities of the recognition system. In the case of the animals being examined, blocking efferent function in the cochlea resulted in reduced frequency resolution capability in the hearing mechanism. Of primary concern to the current discussion is the corrolary to this finding. Since blocking the efferents to the cochlea reduces the frequency discrimination of the hearing mechanism, it is apparent that one significant function of the efferent innervation to the cochlea is to sharpen the frequency discrimination capabilities of the inner ear.

With this information in mind, it is now possible to expand upon Bekesy's (1960, 1962) suggestions relative to the phenomenon of critical bands. The reader will recall Bekesy's conclusion that the critical bands of hearing were too sharp to be adequately explained solely on the basis of the mechanical tuning of the inner ear structures. He postulated a neural inhibition mechanism which would sharpen the frequency resolution capabilities of the inner ear. Recent behavioral research described in detail above indicates that a primary function of the olivo-cochlear bundle is such a frequency sharpening process.

In summary, this section has reviewed the phenomenon of critical bands in hearing. Anatomical and behavioral research has also been reviewed in an attempt to provide a theoretical mechanism for this phenomenon. The proposed theory will now be explained briefly for the reader's convenience. The critical bandwidth mechanism functions in a manner similar to an array of acoustical filters. Auditory stimuli are filtered into narrow bands at the level of the cochlea. The acoustic energy present in each critical band is integrated regardless of where within the given critical band the energy falls. Information as to the level of acoustic energy present in each of the critical bands of the audible spectrum is then passed on to higher auditory centers. Since the mechanical response of the inner ear structures is too gross to provide this fine frequency analysis, a neural inhibition mechanism has been postulated as the mechanism for refining the inner ear's response.

Critical Band Distortion in Sensorineural Hearing Loss

In light of the preceding discussion, it is reasonable to assume that units of the neural inhibitory system of the cochlea would be damaged whenever significant cochlear pathology is present. In such a case one would expect to find wider-than-normal critical bands due to the loss of inhibitory units. Such a phenomenon would give rise to reduced frequency discrimination ability and a deterioration in the ability to recognize signals in background noise as noted in experimental animals with blockage of the olivo-cochlear bundle. Evidence of this phenomenon may be found in limited studies of critical band response with human subjects having hearing loss due to cochlear pathology (deBoer, 1961; Scharf and Hellman, 1966; deBoer and Bouwmeester, 1974, 1976). The condition of widened critical band would result in a greater amount of sensory transducers available for responding to input in any band region affected. Consequently, a given stimulus intensity could elicit a greater neural response from an ear with widened critical bands than from ears with normal critical bands.

The widening of critical bands could be expected to give rise to an abnormally rapid increase in loudness as the level of sound is increased. This is to say that the production of widened critical bands in cochlear injury would give rise to the phenomenon generally referred to as loudness recruitment. The phenomenon of recruitment, however, does not involve any improvement in auditory discrimination because the widening of critical bands reduces the ear's ability to recognize the frequency components of input sounds at the same time that differential loudness sensitivity is increased. This frequency analysis function is essential to the auditory analysis and subsequent understanding of speech sounds (French and Steinberg, 1947; Morton and Carpenter, 1963; Chaves and Scharf 1966; and Scharf, 1970). The phenomenon may, therefore, result in poorer than normal pitch and speech discrimination particularly when communication is carried out in a noisy environment (since more masking noise would be sensed by an ear with widened critical bands). Poor pitch and speech discrimination are, in fact, common symptoms of noise induced hearing loss (Hirsh, 1952; Meurmann, 1954; Butler and Albrite, 1956; Houchins, 1962; O'Neill and Oyer, 1966; Sataloff and Michael, 1973). Within the framework of this model the disruption of speech discrimination ability is dependent upon a process that is relatively independent of hearing threshold acuity. Since the widening of critical bands is due to cochlear changes that do not require changes in the afferent input to the auditory nerve, speech or pitch discrimination may be independent of pure tone hearing threshold loss. The value of the model suggested above is clear when one considers that it has long been recognized that the hearing thresholds are poor predictors of speech discrimination ability. In the particular case of noise induced hearing loss, a further value of this model is that it provides a means for early detection (before threshold changes) of noise susceptibility, and could be effectively incorporated into current hearing conservation practices.

Critical Band Phenomena in Testing Speech Intelligibility

Current theories of audition rely heavily upon the notion of critical bands (e.g., Scharf, 1970). Most simply, a critical band may be conceived as an internal bandpass filter. In the initial conception of critical bands (Fletcher, 1940), the auditory system was seen as consisting of a fixed bank of about 24 critical bands laid end to end, and covering the audible frequency range. The bandwidth of each critical band was seen as a function of its center frequency. More recent accounts have altered this view somewhat in that it is no longer assumed that there is a fixed set of critical bands, but rather, that every audible frequency is surrounded by a critical band. Thus Scharf (1970) has defined the critical band empirically as "that bandwidth at which subjective responses rather abruptly change" (p.159). For example, two stimuli separated in frequency by less than a critical bandwidth will interact in one of a number of ways, while two stimuli separated by more than a critical bandwidth will not.

Critical band mechanisms have been characterized as underlying our ability to process complex acoustic stimuli like speech (Scharf, 1970). The specific task of attempting to measure the critical bandwidth used in the analysis of speech sounds by the auditory system has been indirectly approached in the work of French and Steinberg (1947). These workers determined those frequency-band components of a speech signal that contributes equally to the understanding of that signal. The 20 bands that contribute equally to speech intelligibility in this study compare very well to the parameters of the 24 critical bands found in pure tone psychoacoustic studies. Further support for the underlying contribution of critical band mechanisms to the discrimination of speech sounds comes from a report by Morton and Carpenter (1963). These authors suggested, and found support for, the notion that formants can be identified by listeners even when no prominent energy peak is present as long as the most intense harmonics associated with each formant are separated by at least a critical bandwidth. Similarly, it has been observed that intensity discrimination between two tones is optimal when the tonal separation is about one critical band (Chaves and Scharf, 1966). A related finding was reported by Remez (1977). He presented synthetic vowel stimuli to listeners which varied in terms of the bandwidths of the steady state formants. Subjects in this study noted an abrupt changeover from speech-like to non-speech-like sounds as the formant bandwidth was increased. Although Remez did not report his data in terms of critical band systems, examination of the published data suggest that the speech-non-speech boundary was correlated with the spread of formant energy to within a critical bandwidth. It appears then, that to be heard as speech-like, the synthetic vowel formants had to be separated by at least a critical bandwidth.

In addition to the research on the discrimination of speech signals to normal hearing listeners, the significance of critical band phenomena to speech listening has been noted in research with hearing impaired listeners. Notably, hearing deficits of the sort which may differentially degrade complex signal discrimination without a measureable threshold shift have been characterized as resulting from a widening of criti-bands (deBoer, 1961, 1974; Scharf and Hellman, 1966; deBoer and Bouwmeester, 1974, 1975; Bienvenue et al., 1976, 1978; Bienvenue and Michael, 1977; Bennett et al., 1978).

Scharf (1970) has noted that research findings in this area are limited because most research has relied on filtering systems too broad in frequency bandwidth (i.e., 1/3 octave or wider) for observing critical band phenomena. Present day digital processing techniques may provide sufficient bandwidth control to escape the limitation noted by Scharf. Utilizing discrete Fourier transform techniques on digitized signals, it becomes possible to apply filters of extremely narrow bandwidth and nearly infinite slope to speech stimuli. Thus, many of the questions in this area which have been difficult to address using standard filtering techniques may be examined conveniently via digital processing routines.

To see more clearly how critical band mechanisms influence auditory perception, we may briefly review some recent work in this area. In summarizing work on critical bands we may outline four functional aspects of critical bands which appear to play an important role in the perception of complex stimuli and hence represent fundamental aspects of the hearing aid user's performance. As implied in the work of Fletcher, and many more recent studies (e.g., Zwicker, 1958; Greenwood, 1961), the critical band serves to band-limit background noise. The obvious consequence of this band-limiting is to improve the effective signal-to-noise ratio by allowing only the noise energy within a critical band, centered at the signal frequency, to interfere with the detection of the signal. For example, a hearing aid user may be able to correctly perceive a spoken communication despite background noise simply because much of the energy associated with the noise lies outside the critical bands surrounding the formant frequencies of the speech. A common finding among individuals with cochlear hearing loss (as a result, for instance, with widened critical bands) unfortunately, is that relatively small amounts of background noise are unusually detrimental to speech perception. This phenomena may very well follow directly from the reduced band limiting capabilities of the widened critical bands (Michael and Bienvenue, 1976).

Our ability to discriminate the harmonic content of complex signals (one of the many cues used for instance in speaker identification) is similarly related quite directly to the critical bands phenomenon. Plomp (1964) has demonstrated that listeners are able to discriminate only those partials of a complex tone which lie more than a critical bandwidth apart. If, for instance, a complex tone with a fundamental frequency of 200 Hz is presented, then only about the first six harmonics will be individually detectable because for harmonics above the sixth (1200 Hz) harmonic separation is less than a critical bandwidth (i.e., bandwidth greater than 200 Hz at those frequencies). Clearly cochlear pathology resulting in a widening of critical bands will tend to reduce the number of discriminable harmonics and listeners with this problem will be less able to discriminate signals on the basis of their harmonic content.

A third functional characteristic of critical bands relates to listeners' ability to discriminate phase relations among tone complexes (Scharf, 1970). Phase discrimination appears to play an important role in distinguishing between amplitude and frequency modulation, a type of discrimination which may prove critical for signals such as speech in which changes in amplitude must be distinguished from changes in frequency. In fact, some investigators, notably Ohman (1966) have presented accounts of speech production which are consistent with viewing speech as a simultaneously amplitude- and frequency-modulated signal, while Bunnell (1977) has argued that listeners perceive the syllable timing by demodulating the amplitude modulation characteristics of the acoustic signal.

The fourth functional aspect of critical bands is more general than the above and may well underlie performance in these cases. It is that of frequency sharpening. In the first few milliseconds following the onset of a pure tone, its pitch is relatively indeterminate. As the tone is left on, up to about 200 msec., listeners' pitch judgements improve and then level off at an accuracy which is greater that that predicted on the basis of basilar membrane selectivity alone. This phenomenon has been attributed to an inhibition mechanism which appears to function within critical bands (von Bekesy, 1960). Thus, a portion of our frequency discrimination ability which cannot be attributed to basilar membrane mechanics appears to be due to a frequency sharpening phenomenon which we observe as critical bands.

To summarize, four of the most important functional characteristics of critical bands have been reviewed. In all cases (noise band limiting, harmonic distortion, phase discrimination, and frequency sharpening) it was argued that critical bands play an important role in the correct perception of complex acoustic stimuli. This sort of perception is assumed to underlie the performance of hearing aid users on such tasks as radio, T.V., telephone or noisy conversational listening and hence, the integrity of hearing users' critical bands would appear to represent a limiting factor in their ability to perform these tasks. A widening of critical bands will almost necessarily result in a deficit in performance. Further, as has been suggested, one frequent cause of widened critical bands is exposure to noise. As a consequence of this, the hearing aid user, who is most dependent upon the integrity of his critical band mechanism is also, due to his constant exposure to sound, most susceptible to damage to that mechanism.

In light of the important role in which critical band mechanisms may play in the hearing aid user's listening performance, it is valuable to develop an efficient measure of critical bandwidth for complex signals as an evaluative tool. Such a measure might be particularly valuable if it further incorporated, in the testing situation, stimuli which are closely related to the sorts of stimuli which listeners must actually identify on a daily basis such as speech signals.

Methods for Measuring Critical Bands in Speech Listening

Many techniques for the psychoacoustic measurement of critical bands have been developed. These include critical band measures based upon perceived loudness of complex signals (c.f. Zwicker et al., 1957; Scharf, 1959), narrow band masking effects (c.f. Fletcher, 1940; Greenwood, 1961), the threshold of noise bands when masked by pure tones (c.f. Zwicker, 1954; Greenwood, 1961), the threshold of multitone complexes (c.f. Gassler, 1954), the musical consonance of tone complexes (c.f. Plomp and Levelt, 1962), and tone-on-tone masking effects (Haggard, 1974).

Recent research has concentrated on the development of rapid procedures for the estimation of critical bandwidth (e.g., Haggard, 1974). Several of the traditional psychoacoustic designs are particularly amenable to use in estimating critical bandwidth rapidly. These methods include:

(1) Loudness of Complexes. The loudness of a <u>constant sound pressure level</u>, subcritical, complex signal remains constant as its bandwidth is increased; however, when the signal bandwidth exceeds one critical band the loudness of the signal increases. Using this concept, subjects may be tested by presenting them with a narrowband complex signal and subsequently increasing signal bandwidth without changing the signal's sound pressure level. The subject's critical bandwidth may then be determined by asking the subject to indicate when the signal increases in loudness.

(2) Threshold of Complexes. This design is an extension of the loudness of complexes design. The procedure was originally reported by Gassler (1954). The <u>threshold of a multitone complex</u> (made up of evenly spaced sinusoids) is established. Tones are then added to the complex, increasing the overall bandwidth of the signal, and threshold is reestablished. This procedure is then repeated several times. The critical band may then be determined since the sound pressure level required to elicit threshold sensation remains constant so long as the signal is contained within one critical band. When the overall bandwidth of the signal exceeds one critical band, energy outside the critical band can no longer contribute to the threshold sensation of the complex signal and the sound pressure level for a threshold response increases with the addition of tonal components.

(3) Masking Designs. This design utilized the concept that only that sound energy within one critical band of a given sound signal will contribute to the masking of that signal (Fletcher, 1940). Several methods for the implementation of this design have been evaluated (Greenwood, 1961). Generally, a signal (either a pure tone or a subcritical noise band) is presented embedded within a masking stimulus (either a narrow band of noise or a pair of pure tones). The detectability of the signal is then monitored as a function of masker bandwidth (in the case of the pure tone maskers). Critical bandwidth in this design is defined as the frequency region within which the masker contributes to the masking of the signal (for greater detail see Greenwood, 1961). One masking design that has been reported recently deserves special mention here because it has been propsed as a rapid method for determining critical bandwidth. In this method (Haggard, 1974) the listener is presented with two tones, one serving as a signal, the other as a masker. The frequency separation of the two tones is increased until the listener can resolve the two tones. At this point, it is presumed that the masker tone is outside of the critical band centered on the masked tone. As a result, the masker tone no longer contributes to the masking of the original signal and is now perceived as a second signal.

Also recently, Zwicker (1974) has described a technique for developing what he calls a "psychoacoustical equivalent of tuning curves". The design is essentially a masking technique using a Bekesy audiometer. In this paradigm a listener is presented with two pure tones; one is fixed in level and frequency, the other varies in frequency being produced by the Bekesy audiometer. The variable tone also may be increased or decreased in level by the listener's push-button control. The listener's task is then to adjust the level of the variable tone as it sweeps slowly from 100 Hz to 10,000 Hz so that it just masks the fixed tone. The resultant plot has a remarkable similarity to neural tuning curves recorded from single units in the auditory nerve (c.f. Kiang et al., 1970; Katsuki, 1966; and Evans, 1972). One notable feature of these curves is that as the masking tone approaches the fixed tone, it may be reduced in level and still mask the fixed tone. This is to be anticipated since the masking effectiveness of the variable tone would be proportional to the extent to which it causes stimulation within the critical band region centered at the frequency of

of the fixed tone. The closer the masker gets to the
fixed tone the steeper the function (i.e., the more rapidly its masking effectiveness grows). Although this
method is dependent upon the critical bandwidth phenomenon, it does not give results which are directly inter-
pretable as critical bandwidth information.

An alternative to such laboratory approaches to critical
bandwidth measurement would involve the use of signals which
more closely replicate real-world listening contexts. The
Environmental Acoustics Laboratory (EAL) is currently undertaking this type of approach by using digital processing techniques to develop bandwidth resolution limited speech testing
materials.

A necessary first step is the development of the
software required for varying the bandwidth resolution
of speech. Figure 1 is a block diagram which illustrates
the way in which speech stimuli will be processed for
the proposed experiments. While this figure describes
the signal processing in terms of sets of filters, envelope detectors, modulators, and so forth, it is proposed
that an identical result may be achieved more inexpensive-
ly and with greater versatility and reliability by using
digital signal processing techniques. For digital processing, a computer such as The Pennsylvania State University Electrical Engineering Department's PDP-10 with
analog to digital and digital to analog capabilities may
be used to mimic, at the software level, all of the components illustrated in Figure 1. Thus, prerecorded stimuli may be input to the computer, processed, and then
re-recorded onto audio tape in the processed form.

The stated objective of the stimulus processing procedure is to obtain a set of stimuli which vary in their
frequency resolution. As may be seen from Figure 1, the
proposed processing procedure will achieve this objective simply by varying the band pass characteristics of
the set of filters. If the pass band of each filter is
wide and overlaps that of the neighboring filters, frequency resolution of the output signal will be poor,
while a tightly tuned nonoverlapping set of filters
should provide output signals of much finer frequency
resolution. It is this processing procedure, utilizing
variable bandwidth filters which will be used to generate stimuli for the experiments to be described next.

In this first phase of the new EAL research, the
Northwestern University Auditory Test No. 6 (NU#6)

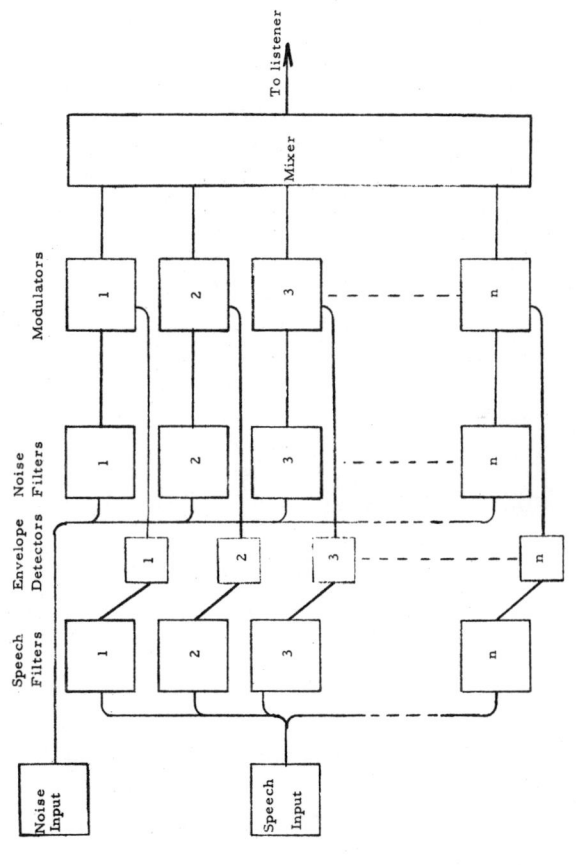

Figure 1. System for generating a variable resolution speech-type signal.

(c.f.Tillman, Carhart and Wilbur, 1963 and Tillman and Carhart, 1966) will be altered by the stimulus processing procedure described above. Subjects selected from the Environmental Acoustics Laboratory trained listener pool will be tested at each of some eight stimulus resolution levels with the NU#6. Two factors will be important in this data: 1) the stimulus resolution condition for which the NU#6 speech discrimination scores of normal hearing subjects first begin to drop; and 2) the rate at which they continue to decline with successive broadening of the stimulus resolution bandwidth. It is anticipated that performance scores will be relatively stable for the first three resolution conditions (resolution bandwidth smaller than or equal to the normal critical bandwidth) and decline rapidly as the resolution bandwidth is broadened beyond the normal critical bandwidth with the remaining five stimulus sets (see Figure 2).

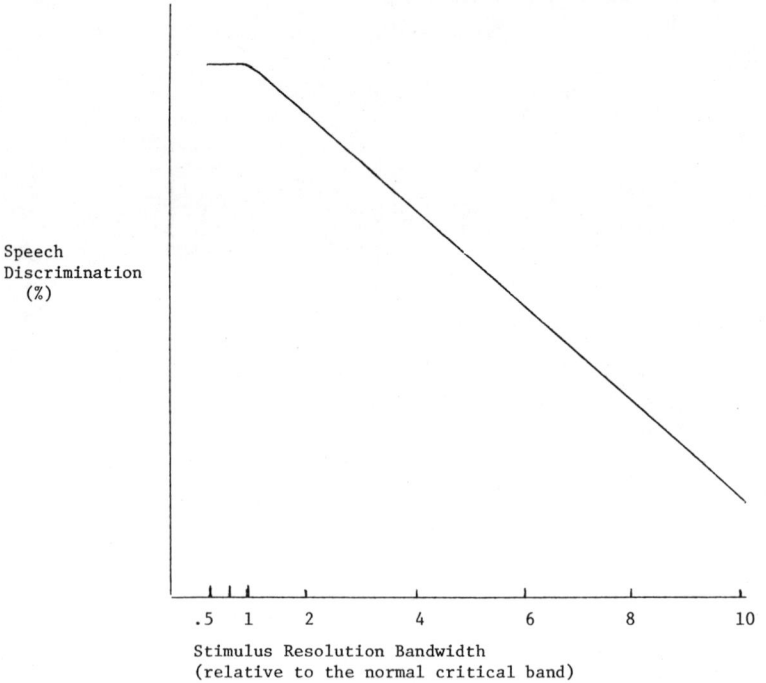

Figure 2. Anticipated performance of normal hearing trained listeners on the speech discrimination task for varying conditions of stimulus resolution bandwidth limitations.

Finally, the digital processing routines which must be developed to achieve the primary goal of the proposed research open up the possibility of examining, as a secondary goal, a wide range of phenomena of a more theoretical nature regarding the relationship between critical bands and the perception of complex stimuli. Of particular interest in this area is the question of the relationships of the frequency and amplitude modulation components of speech to critical band mechanisms. For instance, recent findings suggest that vowel perception in speech may be related to suprasegmental variations in the frequency content of the signal (Strange et al., 1977), but to date no attempt has been made to relate this to the long term frequency resolving power of the listener. Also of interest is the feasibility of applying testing procedures to the identification of individuals especially suited to skilled listening tasks.

Implications and Significance of Critical Bandwidth Testing for Speech

As stated, the principle goal of the new EAL research is the development of an efficient research tool for measuring critical bandwidth within the context of the sorts of stimuli which appear to be most disrupted by signal or by listener distortions (i.e., complex stimuli such as speech). Standard laboratory procedures for measuring critical bandwidth typically involve lengthy psychophysical techniques performed on trained subjects with signals that do not replicate real-world listening tasks (e.g., Fletcher, 1940; Zwicker, 1954; Greenwood, 1961; Haggard, 1974). These procedures, while extremely powerful and accurate, are not easily applied to the evaluation of complex real-world stimuli where listeners are untrained and unwilling to spend many hours listening to, for example, pure tones masked by noise (Fletcher, 1940). By contrast, useful clinical tests such as the NU-Auditory #6 which appears to tap critical bandwidth information, do so without providing any actual bandwidth information. It is felt that the new EAL research will result in a testing procedure which, by merit of the fact that critical bandwidth is directly assessed, would prove especially sensitive in the evaluation of speech listening contexts and may result in the ultimate development of new clinical hearing testing materials which are especially useful in assessing hearing impaired listeners for hearing aid fittings.

Inherent in the signal processing procedures for the proposed research, is the assumption that the reduced frequency resolution of processed stimuli mimics or is analogous to the decrease in auditory frequency resolution resulting from critical band widening. Because of this, the computer program which processes the stimuli may be thought of as a <u>weak</u> analog in the sense that it produces what is believed to be the same sort of decreased frequency resolution found for widening critical bands, but it arrives at this decreased resolution through a process which is not believed to be identical to cochlear auditory processing. Villchur (1977) has commented anecdotally on a processing system he designed which is strikingly similar to that proposed in Figure 1. According to Villchur's report, speech stimuli processed at various levels of frequency resolution are degraded in a manner similar to degradation due to critical band widening; they sound harsh but understandable at narrow bandwidths and become uninterpretable as the bandwidth is widened. Vilchur also points out, however, that this process differs in some ways from cochlear critical band mechanisms. Whether the proposed processing program is or is not precisely analogous to auditory processing may well not seriously affect the validity of the research tools to be developed, but it is one of the principle advantages of using digital signal processing that, should it be necessary to make the program more like a model of the cochlea, such changes could be made with relative ease. Information developed from the use of these materials in the modelling of cochlear pathology could lead to clues in improving the design of hearing aids.

In summary, the new EAL, resolution-limited, speech discrimination materials, because they are directly attuned to a primary mode of auditory signal analysis (the critical band mechanism) and because they will employ the complex, speech stimuli that listeners must analyze in everyday life, should be especially useful in studying aspects of speech listening. The data developed in the initial stages of the new EAL research will elucidate our present understanding of auditory speech processing because it is a type of information not heretofore available. By the use of digital processing techniques it will be possible to identify the contribution to speech discrimination of acoustical information distributed between critical bands. This clarified demonstration of the place held by critical bands in the auditory analysis of complex signals such as speech will provide a basis for precise modelling of speech listening contexts and extend our capabilities in predicting the intelligibility of speech under specified environmental conditions. In addition to the information on auditory speech analysis the new EAL research will provide a new research tool for the study of speech intelligibility and will, thereby, open a new avenue for research on basic phenomena in speech perception.

The final stage of the new EAL research will expand the basis speech discrimination findings into the realm of speech perception in listeners with sensorineural loss of cochlear origin. This is an especially important area for study because this type of hearing loss generally demonstrates a particular tendency towards the deterioration of speech-discrimination in the affected listener. Finally, the research plan would lay the ground work for developing a clinically applicable test for evaluating speech discrimination losses as they relate to critical bandwidth integrity. While existing data on this topic is scanty at present, it appears likely that critical bandwidth losses may be closely related to losses in auditory speech discrimination ability.

References

Bekesy, G. von, Experiments in Hearing. New York: McGraw-Hill, (1960).

Bekesy, G. con, Neural inhibitory units of the eye and skin. Quantitative description of contrast phenomena. J. Opt. Soc. Amer, 50, 1060-1070, (1960).

Bekesy, G. von, Lateral inhibition of hear sensations on the skin, J. Appl. Physiol. 17, 1003-1008, (1962).

Bennett, T., Bienvenue, G., Anthony, A. and Michael, P., Procedures for characterizing certain effects of prolonged noise exposure, J.Acoust. Soc. Amer., 63, suppl. 1, 62, (1978).

Bienvenue, G., Carito, A. and Michael, P., The effects of a variety of noise exposures on A battery of hearing tests. J. Acous. Soc. Amer. 63, Suppl. 1, 64, (1978).

Bienvenue, G., Michael, P. and Violon-Singer, J., The effects of high level sound exposure on the loudness difference limen. Am. Ind. Hyg. Assoc. J., 37, 6280635 (1976).

Bienvenue, G. and Michael, P., The temporary effects of short term noise exposure on masking phenomena., Unpublished EAL research project (1977).

Bienvenue, G., Violon-Singer, J. and Michael, P., Loudness Discrimination Index (LDI): A test for the early detection of noise susceptible individuals., Am. Ind. Hyg. Assoc. J., (1977)

deBoer, E., Measurement of the critical bandwidth in cases of perception deafness. Proc. III Int. Cong. Acoust., 1, 100-103, Elsevier, Amsterdam (1961).

deBoer, E. and Bouwmeester, J., Critical Bands and sensorineural hearing loss. Audiology, 13, 236-259 (1974).

deBoer, E. and Bouwmeester, J., Clinical psychophysics, Audiology, 14, 274-299 (1975).

Bunnell, H.T., Perceiving the temporal structure of amplitude modulated stimuli. Unpublished Master's Thesis. (1978).

Butler, R. and Albrite, J., Arch. Otolar., 63, 411-418 (1956)

Capps, M.J. and Ades, H.W., Auditory frequency discrimination after transection of the Olivo-Cochlear bundle in squirrel monkeys. Esp. Neurel. 21, 141 (1968).

Chaves, J. and Scharf, B., Critical bands and the discrimination of intensity relations in two-tone com-lexes, J. Acous. Soc. Amer., 39, 1262A, (1966).

Dewson, J.H., III., Efferent olivo-cochlear bundle: Some relationships to stimulus discrimination in noise., J. Neurophysiol., 31, 122 (1968).

Dix, M., Observations upon the nerve fiber deafness of multiple sclerosis with particular reference to the phenomenon of loudness recruitment., J. Laryngol., 79, 695 (1965).

Eby, L. and Williams, H., Recruitment of loudness in the differential diagnosis of end organ and nerve fiber deafness. Laryngoscope, 61, 400-414 (1951).

Fex, H., The olivocochlear feedback systems, 77-87, in Sensorineural Hearing Processes and Disorders, A.B. Graham, ed., Little, Brown and Co., Boston, (1967).

Fletcher, H., Auditory patterns, Rev. Med. Phys., 12, 47-65 (1940).

Fowler, E.P., A method for the early detection of otosclerosis., Arch. Otolar., 24, 731-741 (1936).

Fowler, E.P., Marked deafened areas in normal ears,. Arch. Otolar., 8, 151-155 (1928).

Fowler, E.P., The use of threshold and louder sounds in clinical diagnosis., Laryngoscope, 48, 573-588 (1938).

Fowler, E.P., The diagnosis of diseases of the neural mechanism of hearing by the aid of sounds well above threshold. Trans. Am. Otol. Soc., 27. 207-220 (1937).

Fowler, E.P., Loudness recruitment., Arch. Otolar., 78, 749-753 (1963).

French and Steinberg, Factors governing the intelligibility of speech sounds., J. Acous. Soc. Am., 90-119 (1947)

Gassler, G., Uber die horschwelle fur schallereignisse mit verschieden beitem frequenzspektrum., Acustica, 4, 408-414 (1954).

Greenwood, D., Auditory masking and the critical band. J. Acous. Soc. Am., 33, 484-502 (1961).

Haggard, M., Feasibility of rapid critical bandwidth measurements., J. Acous. Soc. Am., 55, 304-308 (1974).

Harris, J.D., A brief critical review of loudness recruitment. Psychol. Bull., 50, 190-203 (1953).

Hirsh, I.J., The Measurement of Hearing. McGraw-Hill Co., New York, Ch. 5 and 11, (1952).

Houchins, R., Volta Rev., 64, 424-426 (1962).

Luscher, E., The difference limen of intensity variations of pure tones and its diagnostic significance., Proc. Roy. Soc. Med., 43, 1116-1128 (1950).

Meurmann, O., Acta Otolar., Suppl. 118, 144-155 (1954).

Michael, P. and Bienvenue, G., A procedure for the early detection of noise susceptible individuals., Am. Ind. Hyg. Assoc. J., 52-55 (1976).

Michael, P., Bienvenue, G., Carito, A. and Prout, J., Early detection of noise induced hearing impairment., Final report to Environmental Protection Agency, Contract No. 68-01-4498 (1978).

Morton, J. and Carpenter, A., Experiments relating to the perception of formants., J. Acous. Soc. Am., 35, 475-480 (1963).

Mygind, S., Ein versuch zur Erklarung des sogenannten regression phanomens (recruitment)., Z. Laryngol. Rhinol., 29, 277-285 (1950).

O'Neill, J. and Oyer, H., Applied Audiometry. New York, Dodd, Mead and Co. 1966.

Olman, S.E.G., Coarticulation in VCV utterances: Spectrographic measurements., J. Acous. Soc.Am., 39, 151-168 (1966).

Pickles, O. and Comis, S.D., Role of centrifugal pathways to cochlear nucleus in detection of signals in noise., J. Neurophysiol., 36, 173-177 (1978).

Plomp, R., The ear as a frequency analyzer., J. Acous. Soc. Am., 36, 1628-1636 (1964).

Plomp, R. and Levelt, W.J.M., Tonal consinance and critical bandwidth., Proc. IV Int. Cong. Acous., Copenhagen (1962)

Rasmussen, G.L., An efferent cochlear bundle., Anat. Rec., 82, 441 (1942).

Remez, R.E., Adaptation of the category boundary between speech and nonspeech: A case against feature detectors., Haskins Laboratories: Status Report on Speech Research SR-50, 151-157 (1977).

Sataloff, J. and Michael, P., Hearing Conservation., C.C. Thomas, Springfield, Ch. 5, (1973).

Scharf, B., Critical bands and the loudness of complex sounds near threshold., J. Acous. Soc. Am., 31, 365-370 (1959).

Scharf, B., Critical bands., In J. Tobias (Ed.), Foundations of Modern Auditory Theory., New York, Academic Press, 1970

Scharf, B. and Hellman, R., A model of loudness summation applied to impaired ears., J. Acous. Soc. Am., 40, 71-78 (1966).

Strange, W., Jenkins, J. and Edman, T., The identification of vowels in vowel-less syllables., J. Acous. Soc. Am., 61, S39 (1977).

Tillamn, T.W. and Carhart, R., An expanded test for speech discrimination utilizing CNC monosyllabic words (Northwestern University Auditory Test No. 6)., Technical Report, SAM-TR-66-55, USAF School of Aerospace Medicine, Aerospace Medical Division (AFSC), Brooks Air Force Base, Texas (1966).

Tillamn, T.W., Carhart, R. and Wilber, L.A., A test for Speech Discrimination composed of CNC monosyllabic words (Northwestern University Auditory Test No. 4), Technical Report SAM-TDR-62-135, USAF School of Aerospace Medicine, Aerospace Medical Division, (AFSC), Brooks Air Force Base, Texas, (1963).

Trahiotis, C. and Elliott, D.N., Behavioral investigations of some possible effects of sectioning the crossed olivocochlear bundle., J. Acous. Soc. Am., 47, 592 (1970).

Villchur, E., Electronic models to simulate the effect of sensory distortions on speech perception by the deaf., J. Acous. Soc. Am., 62, 665-674 (1977).

Zwicker, E., Die verdecklung von schmalbandgerauschen durch sinustone., Acoustica, 4, 415-420 (1954).

Zwicker, E., Ueber pdychologische und methodische grundlagen der lautheit., Acoustica, 8, 237-258 (1958).

Zwicker, E., Flottorp, G. and Stevens, S.S., Critical bandwidth in loudness summation., J. Acous. Soc. Am., 29, 548-557 (1957).

Chapter 8

Digital Approaches to Auditory Training

Harris Drucker, Ph.D.

Introduction

In the past ten years we have seen a revolution in digital technology allowing us to perform old functions in a new way or allowing the introduction of new techniques that could not be done using the old technology. An example of the old done in a new way is the calculator, formerly a table top mechanical kluge that had to be plugged into a 120 volt eletrical socket. Now we have hand held calculators with nine volt batteries that can be obtained for $10.00. At the high end of the calculator market we have programmable calculators that for hundreds of dollars equal or surpass the computing power of the original electronic digital computers that might have cost hundreds of thousands of dollars. An example of the new is the electronic fuel system on some of the more expensive cars which allows precise control of fuel/air mixture and other variables for optimum performance. Sensors record air temperature, engine temperature, and engine speed and pass these to a computer that adjusts the variables to obtain the best fuel economy. Also available are the new electronic games that ten years ago would be impossible.

The technology that has allowed us to do this is called LSI, short for large scale integration. In LSI, the eqivalent of ten thousand transistors or more are deposited on a chip of silicon that might be only half a square millimeter in area. The cost of producing the first LSI chip that performs the simplest functions is fabulously expensive, anywhere from a hundred thousand dollars to a million dollars. First an electrical schematic has to be produced that is thousands

of times normal size. Then this is made into a mask, somewhat
similar to a photographic negative that will be the same size
as the eventual LSI chip. A chip of silicon is exposed in
somewhat the same fashion as a photographic print is exposed
through a negative. However, in the chip of silicon we deposit conducting materials rather than a photographic subject.
This process takes place in what we termed "clean rooms" so
that tiny particles of dust do not inadvertently get deposited
on the chip. On the size scale we are talking about here,
the particle of dust that would be visible to the maked eye
will completely destroy the chip. Various manufacturing defects including impurities in the original silicon wafer, dust
and problems in bonding eternal leads to the chip means that
many of the chips we produce are defective. Defective chips
cannot be repaired, so they are junked, lowering the yield
and driving up the manufacturing costs. In spite of the fact
that the original costs are so high, the production of millions of these chips results in a cost per chip that is very
low, sometimes as low as thirty cents for these chips that
perform the simplest functions to twenty dollars for chips
that are the heart of the micro-computer. Later we will show
how these digital chips can be used in an auditory trainer.
However, first we must discuss how to convert speech into a
form that is internally compatible with these chips.

Analog-to-Digital Conversion

The human race uses the decimal system to count, multiply, add, subtract, and divide using the ten decimal digits
(decimal derives from the Latin, meaning ten). Electronically
we find it easier to use the binary system in decimal logic.
Binary and digital have come to mean essentially the same
thing -- two states. Electronically the two states are Off
and On. Thus we might count:
     Off for Decimal 0
     On for Decimal 1
How do we count higher now that we have used up the two binary digits? Namely, just the same as we do in decimal after
we have used the digits 0 through 9 -- put a 1 in the tens
column and start the ones column again.
     On Off for decimal 2
     On On for decimal 3
It gets rather cumbersome using Off and On notation. Thus
for convenience, we use a shorthand notation, a "1" for an
"On" and a "0" for an "Off". Thus to count in binary we
would go:

Digital Approaches to Auditory Training

000_2 0_{10}
001_2 1_{10}
010_2 2_{10}
011_2 3_{10}
100_2 4_{10}
101_2 5_{10}
110_2 6_{10}
111_2 7_{10}

You see that I have used a subscript two by the binary numbers to indicate base two. One must be careful because obviously 111_{10} is a much larger number than 111_2. Using binary digits (or bits) is much more cumbersome because it takes up so many more bits to represent a number than using decimal digits. With:

     One bit we can represent two numbers ($0_{10}, \rightarrow 1_{10}$)
     Two bits we can represent four numbers ($0_{10} \rightarrow 3_{10}$)
     Three bits we can represent eight numbers ($0_{10} \rightarrow 7_{10}$)
     Four bits we can represent sixteen numbers ($0_{10} \rightarrow 15_{10}$)
     n bits we can represent 2^n numbers ($0_{10} \rightarrow 2^n-1$).

Bit is a contraction for "binary digit".

One of the problems we must overcome is the fact that the speech waveform is continuous while digital logic is not. Look at a typical speech waveform -- the amplitude at any time is a particualr voltage that may be specified as accurately as you need.(Figure 1). Therefore at time to the voltage may be 2.762 volts and in general the voltage at any time may be one of an infinite set ranging from 0 to 4 volts. Suppose now internal to the computer I use two bit numbers to represent four possible values, then I can only represent the discrete values; 0, 1, 2 and 3. Therefore I cannot represent 2.762 volts. To represent the analog waveform internally, we sample the analog waveform with the following conventions.

Analog	Digital Representation
0 to 1 volts	00
1 to 2 volts	01
2 to 3 volts	10
3 to 4 volts	11

The replacement of a continuum of values with discrete values is called quantization (Schwartz, 1970; Hankin, 1978). The whole process of sampling and quantization is called analog to digital conversion (ADC). How often must we sample? The answer is -- at least twice the highest frequency so that speech limited to 10 KHz must be sampled at least 20,000 samples/sec. The ADC converts an analog signal to a digital signal so that we may do such digital manipulations as filtering. Suppose we ignore this processing step for the time being and take the ADC output and convert it right back to an analog

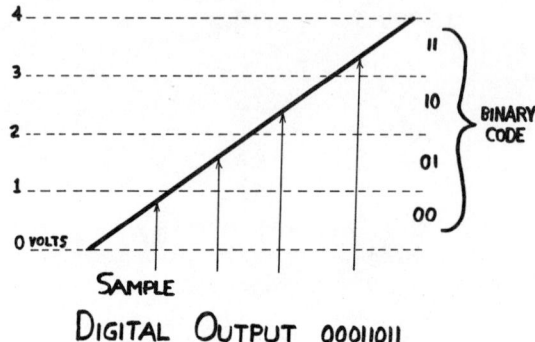

Figure 1. Example of quantizing analog values in the analog to digital conversion process. At the sampling times represented by the arrows, analog values are replaced with binary codes.

waveform for presentation to our listener. This is done by a DAC (digital to analog converter). What we should be able to do is reproduce the hypothetical ramp waveform. The first four samples of the waveform are 00, 01, 10, and 11. What are the four outputs of the DAC to be? Unfortunately the 00 could have easily come from a sample value of .9 volts as well as from .2 volts. We thus arbitrarily decide that the DAC output voltages should correspond to:

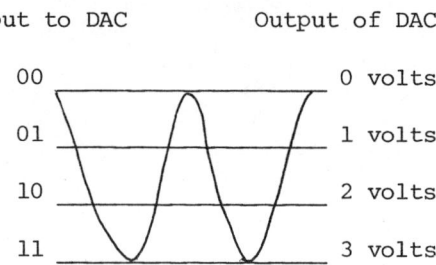

Thus the DAC output does not look like the original input (Figure 2). This irretrievable loss of information is due to the quantization process and in this case causes a maximum 1 volt error difference between the original input and the output. We can smooth the waveform somewhat by low pass filtering but we cannot recover the lost information. Of course ordinarily we would not A/D convert and then immediately D/A convert. Whatever processing is done digitally (Figure 3), the quantization process causes a loss in information. Strangely enough, as bad as two bit (four level) speech

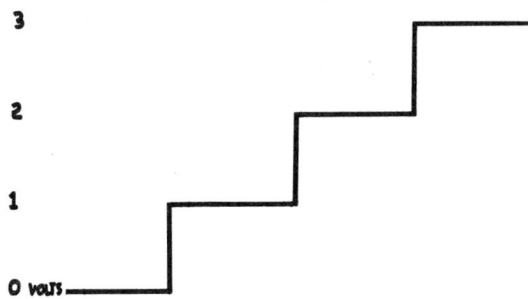

Figure 2. DAC output due to binary input 00011011 caused by waveform of Figure 1.

sounds, it is highly intelligible. In fact in a classic set of experiments by Licklider (1947), it was shown that two level speech (one bit representation) was highly intelligible if the speech was first high pass filtered before being quantized to two levels (Figure 4). As might be expected, the resultant speech does not sound very natural. To increase the naturalness of the speech we can increase the number of bits. Suppose we divide the 0 to 4 volt range into eight parts using three bits.

Figure 3. Digital Speech Processing System.

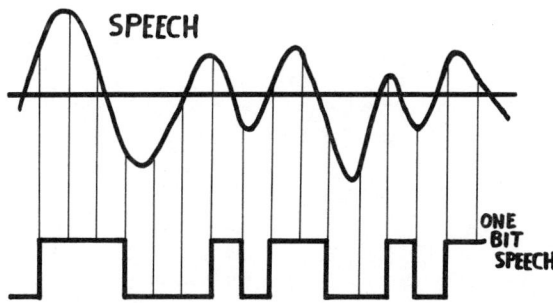

Figure 4. Speech digitized to two levels (one bit speech).

Analog	Output of ADC
0.0 to 0.5 volts	000
0.5 to 1.0 "	001
1.0 to 1.5 "	010
1.5 to 2.0 "	011
2.0 to 2.5 "	100
2.5 to 3.0 "	101
3.0 to 3.5 "	110
3.5 to 4.0 "	111

The maximum quantization error is .0 volts, half of what it was with the two bit representation. Eight bit (256 steps) representation can hardly be distinguished from the real thing. With eight bits, the maximum quantization error for a 4 volt input is

$$q = \frac{4 \text{ volts}}{2^8} = \frac{4}{256} = \frac{1}{64} \text{ volt}$$

The questions now arise: Can we do the "old", namely analog speech processing without using the conventional analog digital circuitry with some advantage and can anything new be done that could not be done before? (Gold, 1977; Jaynant, 1976).

There are a few critical terms that must be defined here: Real time processing-output rate equals input rate with no time delay. Real time processing is necessary for practical hearing aids.

Non-real time processing- processing time is slower than the input rate. The input data is stored, processed at a slower speed and then transmitted to the output at a later time.

Digital processing - a processing approach that is implemented in two-state electronics.

Computer processing - a form of digital processing where the processing is encoded in the form of a stored computer program that manipulates the data. Often termed software processing, computer processing is flexible because programs can be modified to try different processing techniques.

Hardware processing - digital processing which is all hardware. The hardware approach is faster than the software approach and is thus more likely to be used in real time processing, however, it is not as flexible as software.

How fast must a computer be to process raw speech? If

one assumes a speech signal bandlimited to 6 KHz, then the sampling theorem tells us to sample this signal 12,000 times per second. To get a better representation, we usually sample much faster - let us assume 20,000 samples/second. Now let us assume a modest sized program to manipulate the data - say 1000 instructions. The program must go through these instructions 20,000/second for real time operation, equivalent to a computing speed of twenty million instructions per second, a rate far higher than available with presently available microcomputers. Thus we cannot expect sophisticated real time processing techniques with the same small computers that run your video games or control your car. In postauricular or body aids we also have the problems of high voltage (5 volts) and higher (than conventional aid) current.

Can hardware realizations be constructed that implement sophisticated algorithms in real time? The answer is yes but recall that the hardware approach is not very flexible and the economics of the marketplace demand that there be enough users to produce a low cost per electronic chip. All the hearing impaired cannot use an identical processing scheme and hence it is unlikely that the construction of special purpose integrated circuits can be justified.

The problem we are trying to solve is to make speech more intelligible for those persons with sensorineural hearing loss typified by high frequency recruitment, raised thresholds and a consequent loss of dynamic range. Shown in Figure 5 are hypothetical thresholds and discomfort levels for a typical patient as compared to a normal listener. The discomfort level has not changed much but we have a severely elevated threshold. The difference in dB between discomfort and threshold is called the dynamic range and one of the basic problems for the hearing impaired is that the dynamic range of the speech exceeds that of the ear's to perceive it. We have superimposed the range of conversational speech on this figure (Dunn and White, 1938). Using conventional circuit techniques we can amplify the incoming speech -- this has the effect of raising both extremes of conversational speech by the same amount (the gain). Through filtering, or equalization, we can affect both extremes in the same manner. We cannot, using gain or equalization, change the dynamic range. This causes problems to the hearing aid user. If he raises the hearing aid's volume so that the least perceivable sounds are above threshold, then the loud sounds exceed discomfort.

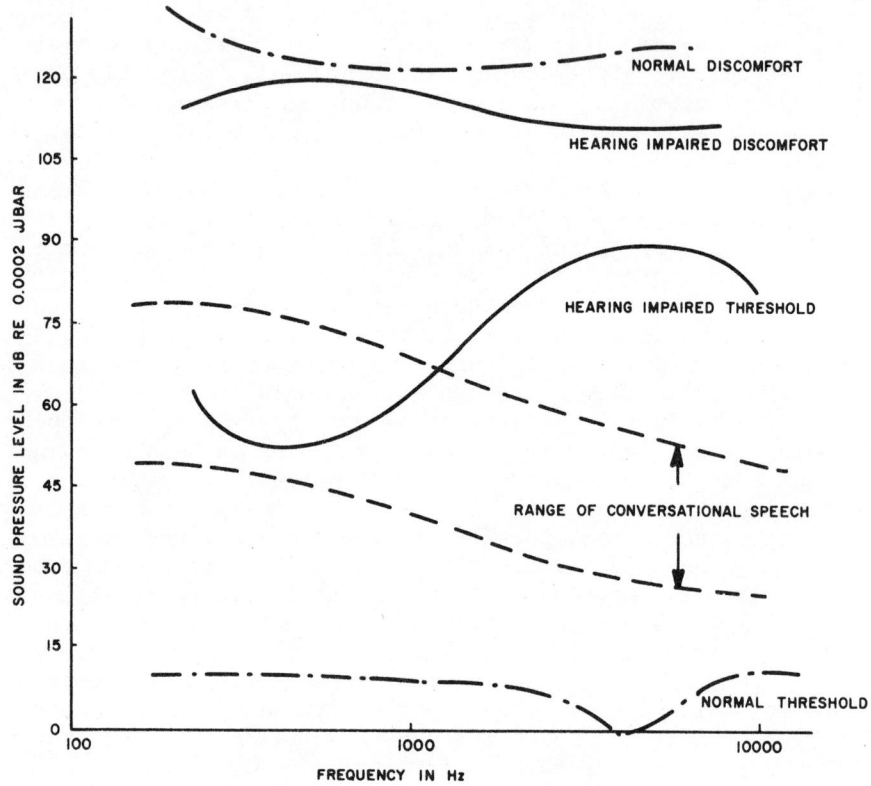

Figure 5. Threshold-discomfort levels for hearing impaired subject and normal subject. Superimposed is the approximate range of conversational speech.

On the other hand, if the volume is lowered so discomfort is not exceeded, then those sounds lowest in intensity may not exceed threshold. What we need to do is alter the dynamic range of speech so that it fits into the listener's dynamic range. This can be accomplished with a compressor (Figure 6). Also shown is the input-output characteristics of the normal amplifier with a slope of one. Raising the gain raises the curve but does not change the slope. Therefore, a 50 dB input dynamic range translates into a 50 dB output dynamic range for the normal amplifier. For the compressor with a slope of .5, an input dynamic range of 50 dB translates into a 25 dB output range. By following the compressor with an ordinary amplifier, we can move this range to any absolute level, examples: 50 to 75 dB SPL or 75 to 100 dB SPL. In a sense, compressors make loud sounds softer and soft sounds

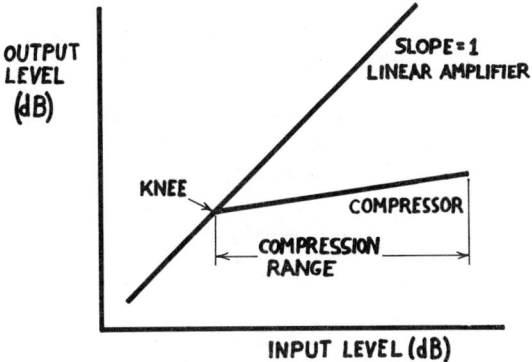

Figure 6. Input-output compressor characteristics.

louder. Again using the .5 slope example, we see that a 20dB increase at the input which is a 100 to 1 increase in power becomes a 10 dB or a 10 to 1 power increase instead of the larger 100 to 1 increase at the output of the ordinary amplifier. On the other hand, a 100 to 1 decrease becomes instead a 10 to 1 decrease. In making soft sounds louder, we want to make sure that the low level background noise is not brought above threshold. For this reason, we put a threshold "knee" in the curve below which the slope is 1 or greater. If the slope is greater than 1, the soft background noise falls off faster than it ordinarily would.

In Figure 7 we show a plot of gain (output minus input) vs. input level. The gain decreases as we increase the input signal level once we pass the threshold "knee". However, we do not instantaneously change the gain as the input signal level varies -- this would destroy the ordinary dynamics of speech. What we want to do is compress almost instantaneously on fast large transitions (within a short time called the

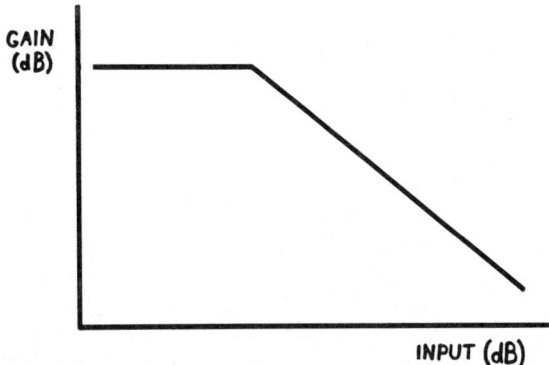

Figure 7. Input-gain compressor characteristics.

attack time) so that the gain is reduced and slowly increase the gain as the waveform amplitude decreases (termed the release time). We have found a 1 msec. attack time and a 20 msec. release time to be reasonable. If the release time is too long, weak consonants following strong vowels, which is very typical of speech, are not amplified enough (Figure 8).

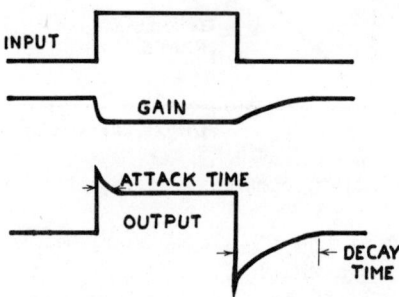

Figure 8. Definition of attack and release times.

What compression ratio (slope) should be used? Ideally

$$\text{Compression Ratio} = \frac{\text{Perceived Dynamic Range}}{\text{Dynamic Range of Speech}}$$

However, the compression ratio would then be a function of frequency. For the hypothetical case we presented before, we need larger compression at the higher frequencies. It should be pointed out that the characteristics of the compressor we are describing are those of the analog compressor -- digital implementation may cause different characteristics.

Compression Using Nonuniform Quantization

In trying to decrease the dynamic range of the speech waveform, we find that digital encoding of speech inherently performs this purpose. For instance, a two bit digital waveform with a 4 level capability has a $20 \log \frac{4}{1} = 12\text{dB}$ dynamic range no matter what the input dynamic range. However, two bit speech though intelligible to the normal hearing probably would not be acceptable to the hearing impaired. Furthermore, it is very unpleasant to listen to, therefore fatiguing just because of its discrete nature and the noise problem. Any noise, no matter how small, is raised to the first quantized level, therefore lowering the dynamic range. Eight bit representation sounds fairly natural, with 256 levels and a 20 log 256 or 48dB dynamic range. For those individuals with a dynamic range of less than 48 dB, we can use nonuniform quantization (Figure 9). In this figure, I have indicated only four quantization levels for clarity purposes. By nonuniform quantization, we mean that the step size is different for different regions. Where the signal tends to be large, the step size tends to be gross; where the signal is small, we use finer quantization sizes. You see that the dynamic range has been compressed. In using 8 bit quantization which is 128 levels, we would want to make the higher levels nonuniform but have uniform quantization at lower levels in order not to destroy the dynamics of the speech at lower levels. In actual practice, we would also high pass filter to emphasize the higher frequencies.

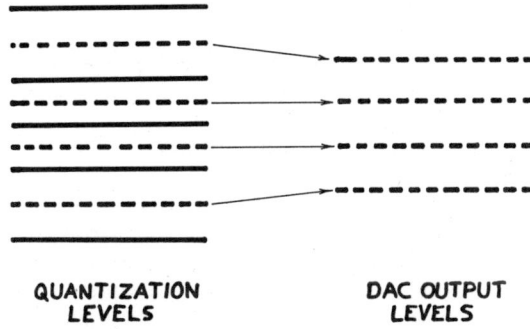

Figure 9. Nonlinear quantization.

Delta Modulation

Delta modulation is an old technique (Panter, 1965; Winkler, 1963) used for transmitting speech. It is not too popular these days because it has a limited dynamic range, especially at high frequencies. Thus it might be perfect for our hypothetical patient with high frequency sensorineural loss. The basic model of the system consists of a comparitor and an integrating network (Figure 10). The comparitor compares the speech input to the output of the integrator. If the speech signal is greater than the integrator output, the comparitor output is a positive pulse, otherwise a negative pulse. The integrator is merely a charge storage device. When the comparitor output is positive, the output goes up, otherwise down. In Figure 11, I have overlaid the audio signal on top of the integrator output. If the integrator out-

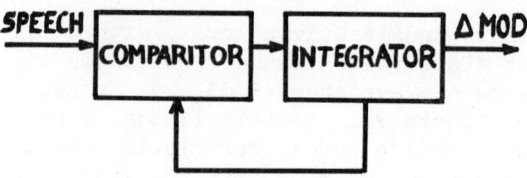

Figure 10. Delta modulation.

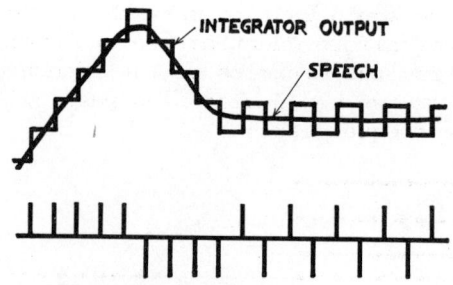

Figure 11. Delta modulation waveforms.

put goes too high the comparitor outputs negative pulses driving the integrator output in the other direction.

The problem with delta modulation comes from what is termed slope overload. The integrated signal can change only a step size at a time. Therefore, if the audio signal changes too fast, the integrated signal cannot follow the audio (Figure 12). The problem gets worse the higher the amplitude and the higher the frequency because the higher the frequency the less time there is to reach the maximum amplitude and the larger the amplitude the more steps must be taken to reach this amplitude. Suppose σ is the step size and we can sample every T_s seconds. The maximum slope is the σ/T_s volts/sec. or σf_s where $f_s = 1/T_s$. The slope of a triangle wave that goes from 0 to A_{max} in T seconds is

$$\frac{A_{max}}{T} = \sigma f_s \qquad A_{max} = \sigma f_s T$$

If we think of the triangle wave as having a period of $2T = 1/f$, then

$$T = \frac{1}{2f}$$

$$A_{max} = \frac{\sigma f_s}{2f}$$

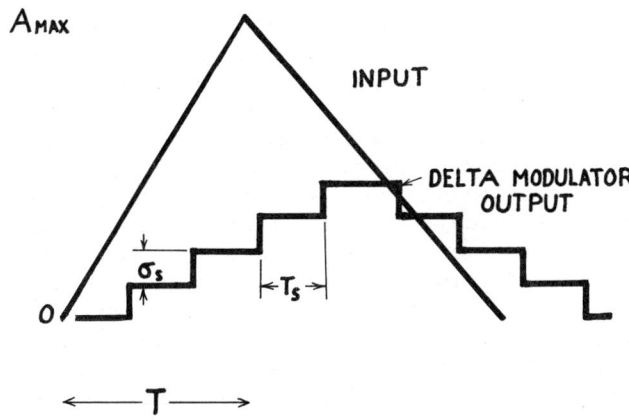

Figure 12. Slope overload in delta modulation.

What this formula states is that the imput amplitude at a certain frequency is greater than A_{max}, the output of the delta modulation will be no greater than A_{max}, thereby reducing the dynamic range. Furthermore, as the frequency increases, A_{max} decreases so that the dynamic range decreases with the increasing frequency. We can make adjustments to the dynamic range by varying the step size σ, f_s or performing filtering because filtering varies A_{max} as a function of frequency. The delta modulation scheme and the nonuniform quantization procedure discussed previously are examples of digital schemes that have no analog counterpart. Delta modulation does not require a digital computer. Furthermore, it can be implemented without digital (+5 volt) logic. Thus, delta modulation could be implemented in a postauricular aid.

A Two Channel System

Previous work has been done on a two channel, all analog compression system (Villchur, 1973; Yanick, 1977, 1976; Yanick and Drucker, 1976). A turnkey two channel version (Figure 13) that is a mixture of analog and digital circuitry is presently being breadboarded by a Master's thesis student. By turnkey we mean that a user, totally unfamiliar with computers can use this computer based trainer. The reason for the two channels is that (a) different compression ratios can be used for the two channels thereby more closely matching the dynamic ranges of the listener at high and low frequencies, and (b) since on the average the low frequency components are high intensity vowels and the high frequency components are

low intensity consonants, the high intensity vowels will not
cause a gain reduction in the system as it would in a one
channel system. Recall that a compressor works by reducing
the gain at high input levels. If a high intensity vowel precedes a low level consonant, the gain would be reduced so
that the consonant would not be amplified to desired levels.
In a two channel system, we are crudely trying to separate
the vowels and consonants so that the high frequency compressor will tend to have larger gain than the low frequency compressor because of the smaller intensity of the high frequency
consonants. In addition, by putting a higher level of gain
into the high frequency channel, we try to insure that the
maximum output levels of both stages are the same, distorting
the relative amplitudes of the consonants and vowels as it
occurs in normal speech but with the approximate idea that
the consonants carry more intelligibility than the vowels and
thus perhaps should be amplified more. The vowel-consonant
division behaving as a low frequency-high frequency separation
is not strictly true of course but the two channel system
does seem to work. Recombination of low and high channels is
followed by equalization. The listener is allowed to vary
the high frequency compression ratio, the low frequency compression ratio, the overall volume and the equalization. The
compressors work over a 30dB (low frequencies) or 36dB (high
frequencies) input dynamic range corresponding to the approximate dynamic range of normal speech.

These compressors are controlled by the output of a DAC
which in turn is controlled by a small computer termed a
microcomputer. The output of the high pass and low pass filters are envelope detected (Figure 14) to get an overall intensity. The microprocessor alternately samples each envelope
detector to get an overall indication of relative intensity.
Knowing the relative intensity, the microcomputer can control

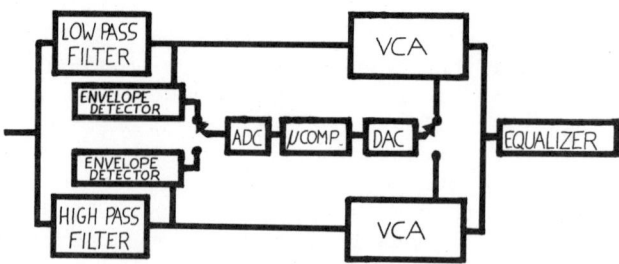

Figure 13. Two channel compression.

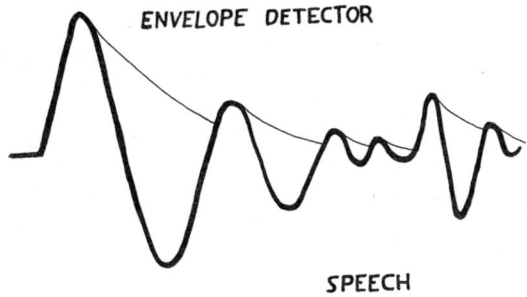

Figure 14. Envelope detector.

the gain of a VCA (voltage controlled amplifier) through a DAC. The control of the gain proceeds in the following manner. If the envelope increases in value, the gain is reduced in direct logarithmetic proportion. As part of the envelope detector is a filter that constrains the change rate to about a millisec./40dB change in the input. If the envelope decreases, the microcomputer increases the gain at a rate of 40dB/20msec. change. In this manner, we account for the desired release time. The advantge of the hybrid (digital and analog) approach over the analog is closer control of compressor characteristics and price.

The reason for the hybrid approach to the two channel compressor is that at the time the breadboard was first being conceived, there was no cheap hardware to perform the digital equivalent of filtering in real time. Filtering in the digital domain is done using multiplication, addition, and subtraction instead of using amplifiers, resistors, and capacitors. These manipulations must however be done in real time so that the output signal goes out at a rate equal to the input rate. Suppose we band limit to 8 KHz, a reasonable value to retain the frequency information although the normal listener can get by with a lot less. Theoretical considerations from communication theory tell us that we must sample at a rate twice this or 16,000 samples/sec. In practice, we must usually go to a much higher sampling rate, perhaps 25,000 samples/sec. This gives the computer 1/25,000 or 40 sec to take each sample, perform the equivalent of high pass filtering and low pass filtering, compute a nonlinear gain, equalize and output data to the DAC. This is an awful lot to do in 40 sec. The microprocessor manufacturers are just starting to come out with the hardware that makes this feasible.

Conclusions

We have shown several different implementation procedures for auditory trainers. They are not applicable to hearing aids because of the large voltage requirements (5 volts) and the large current drain. However, because of the fact that these models can be constructed from LSI chips, they can be constructed at a much lower cost with much better fidelity than hearing aids. We plan to build these devices in the near future and test them.

References

Datel Catalogue, Datel Systems, Inc., 1020 Turnpike Street, Canton, Massachusettes, 02021.
Dunn, H.K. and White, S.D., Statistical measurements on conversational speech, <u>J.Acous.Soc. Amer.</u>, Vol. 11, 278-298 (1938).
Gold, B., Digital speech networks, <u>Proceeding of the IEEE</u>, Vol. 65, No. 12, Dec. (1977).
Hankin, S., <u>Communication Systems</u>, Wiley, (1978).
Jaynant, S., Ed., <u>Waveform Quantization and Coding</u>, IEEE Press, New York, (1976).
Licklider, J.C.R. and Pollack, I., Effects of differentiation integration and infinite peak clipping upon the intelligibility of speech, <u>J. Acous. Soc. Amer.</u>, Vol. 20, 42-51 (1947).
Panter, P.F., <u>Modulation, Noise, and Spectral Analysis</u>, McGraw-Hill, (1965).
Schwartz, M., <u>Information, Transmission, Modulation and Noise</u> McGraw-Hill, (1970) 2nd Ed.
Special Issue on Speech Recognition, <u>IEEE Trans. Acoustics, Speech, and Signal Processing</u>, February, (1975).
Special Issue on Microprocessor Applications, <u>Proc. of the IEEE</u>, February, (1978).
Villchur, E., Signal processing to improve speech intelligibility in perceptive deafness, <u>J. Acous. Soc. Amer.</u>, Vol. 53, 1646-1657 (1973).
Yanick, P., The effects of signal processing on consonant identification for persons with sensorineural hearing loss., <u>J. Soc. Med. Aud.</u>, Vol. 4, No. 4, (1977).
Yanick, P., The effects of signal processing on the intelligibility of speech in noise for subjects possessing sensorineural loss. <u>J. Amer. Aud. Soc.</u>, Vol.2,No.5,1976
Yanick,P. and Drucker,H., Signal processing to improve intelligibility in the presence of noise for persons with ski slope hearing loss. <u>IEEE Trans in ASSP</u>.24:6 507-12 1976.

Chapter 9

Post-Fitting Counseling
of the Hearing Impaired Listener

Steven W. Vargo, Ph.D.

Introduction

In most societies ostensibly referred to as "civilized", auditory-verbal communication is the principal avenue by which man communicates with his society. Ideas are generated and verbalized, intellectually parried, developed and very often honed to a fine concept. The uniqueness of a spoken language is that it possesses an almost unlimited capability for expanding, generating new forms and discarding old ones and modifying those which require some change. Beyond those possibilities, spoken language carries with it information and meanings above its literal definitions. The suprasegmental aspects of speech which include inflection, rhythm patterns and pauses, carry nuances in meaning which transcend and/or embellish the literate. Obviously, such capability is a clear reserve for enriching the subtlety of meaning.

The inability to perceive and/or understand, because of hearing impairment, the literal components of spoken language must substantially diminish the psychosocial behaviors which represent the foundation of human life. Deprivation in whole, or in part, of auditory function, especially during the formative years creates a void of immense proportions which may never be adequately filled. Auditory impairment poses problems and difficulties different than, and similar to, physical disabilities of other types. The ramifications of inadequate auditory function will be viewed from the standpoint of aural rehabilitation procedures, but especially as it relates to the uses and abuses of personal amplification by the individual.

In this paper it is my objective to look at and assess, as well as critically examine, how the hearing-impaired listeners' needs for communication can be improved, remain unchanged, or become worse with the use of amplification. It is also of more than passing interest to discuss social preconceptions of hearing help, family and other group unit interactions and individual coping mechanisms elicited in the deafened. The ultimate purpose of this discussion, however, is to develop in the hearing health worker, be he Audiologist, Otologist, or hearing aid specialist, an improved understanding of the overt and underlying psychosocial pressures and methods by which the hearing impaired-listener can improve his communicative skills. For the professional, it is especially important to understand that self-image, in many cases, is, or can be substantially altered, usually in a negative manner, when the individual is faced with the pressure of using amplification.

Communication Breakdown and Hearing Impairment

The establishment and maintenance of an adequate auditory-verbal communication system is dependent upon the relative integrity of both the auditory mechanism and vocal-integrative processing systems. Because our primary interest is the hearing mechanism, emphasis will be directed toward its dysfunction and consequent ramifications in language.

For the individual born with congenital hearing loss of severe sensorineural type, whatever the etiology, it will probably require that a visual-signing system of communication be learned in order to function in life. The potential of amplification, as an effective provider of auditory information, will have little or no meaning to the severely hearing-impaired listener for everyday needs. At best, personal amplification may provide a severely distorted auditory perceptual pattern whose meanings may only best be described as being virtually devoid of information. Nevertheless, for some individuals, the presence of primitive acoustical signals may serve a useful purpose in alerting one to environmental dangers. On the whole, however, personal amplification tends not to be effectively employed.

Our main interest is with the adult who has matured in his milieu with an intact auditory-verbal communication system, but has begun to experience some progressive degree of sensorineural hearing impairment which has begun to interfere with his economic and social relationships as well as self-image. In general, the individual in his late fifties or early sixties, is well on his way toward completion of a career which is now threatened by a disruption of lifestyle. Because society and self continue to demand productivity in our culture, the resolution of his communicative breakdown due to hearing impairment demands some action on his part.

Somatopsychology and Coping

The influence and relationship of body (somato) changes e.g., amputation, on psychological states of personality and social perceptions is only partially appreciated by the professional community. Most of what is known has been learned from the physically handicapped population, especially military veterans. Much of what we can profitably apply toward hearing impairment must, therefore, be extrapolated from the physical disability studies reported on by Wright (1955) and others. Although differences in theories exist concerning the dynamics of psychosocial interactions and personality change, as well as terminology, there appears to be general agreement on the surface on the mechanisms involved. From childhood onward, but particularly in adolescence, western culture pressures its members to be physically ideal and whole, with spotless grooming and greaseless hair. These fabricated ideals receive reinforcement through the advertising media and obsess society with physical perfection in body. By its very emphasis on wholeness and perfection an attitude of disdain and intolerance surfaces and is directed toward those not fortunate enough to possess good physical integrity. In stark contrast to this wholeness of self, the legless amputee does not require much more to envisage himself as less than worthy of life. Hearing impairment, while not so obvious as a legless body, can also bring forth feelings of hopelessness and depression just as a missing member.

Bender (1964), and Schilder (1964) have proposed theories dealing with body image awareness, and its modifications due to physical disability, which provide some of the most relevant knowledge on the somatopsychology of handicaps. It is known that physical changes, e.g., paralysis, amputation, etc. whether conspicuous or not, create within an individual a constellation of reactions and mental sets which are self-directed, and some which are allo (other world) directed. Some reactions are rational and realistic, while others are delusional and fantasy. In some individuals the intensity of response totally overwhelms the psyche rendering it totally helpless and incapable of self help.

Recognition of less than an adequate wholeness of self is a painful admittance, though not necessarily acceptance of that self-image. The vivid facts are often too intense to confront. Quite often, the characteristic response toward the self is a complete denial of the existence of any physical dysfunction, and if carried far enough is viewed as an obliterative phenomenon which erases and denies inadequacy. Thus, what does not exist, or is conceived not to exist, can be dismissed and considered solved. Assuming, on the other hand, that recognition precedes confrontation, directly or indirectly, and with nuclear family including audiological support, there is good reason to predict acceptance and adjustment to the sensorineural hearing loss and communicative difficulties.

Clearly, auditory impairment does not outwardly call attention to itself, unlike a post-stroke paralysis, and therefore becomes a "silent" disability for most individuals. Because the inability to understand others has, over the centuries, been associated with mental retardation, and because hearing impairment produces a similar, albeit not identical concept, the two disabilities are often mistaken for each other. One has only to research the professional literature in order to discover how often an average intelligent, but deaf youngster, had been committed to state institutions for the retarded for years or an entire lifetime.

Psychosocial Dynamics and Hearing Loss

The individual with physical disability, whether it be hearing impairment, blindness or amputee, is daily obliged to confront himself with his limitations in society. Because auditory impairment is not obvious, its possessor can create and foster an illusory adequacy of communication function under many situations. Thus, the hearing-impaired listener can "fake it" for a long period of time, effectively denying his problems, but constantly waiting anxiously to be caught in his difficulty. The rejection of the recommendation for wearing a hearing aid is a rejection or non-acceptance of the individual's physical problem. With little motivation, the hearing-impaired person can develop some of the most convincing reasons for not using amplification. One of these "crutches" often observed is Projection. In this psychosocial construct, the hearing-impaired person projects his communicative inadequacy as being caused by others. In this concept it is the speaker who fails to enunciate clearly or otherwise speaks so poorly that no one can understand what has been said. Until others improve their speaking patterns, there is little or nothing he can do to improve the listening situation.

One of the markedly drastic responses in coping with the frustrations brought about by auditory impairment is Withdrawal. This constuct represents a form of escapism from the realities of everyday psychosocial communicative situations which cannot be otherwise managed. More often than not withdrawal represents a cumulative reaction to repeated difficulties and failures to achieve adequate social intercourse. Characteristically, this mechanism of non-coping has been associated with the aged who have traditionally been viewed as inflexible types. Withdrawal, however, can be observed in youngsters who have not found social acceptance in school and/or at play. In the presence of marginally acceptable social situations, the hearing-impaired child is generally excluded from group activities unless extraordinary efforts are made to bring him into the mainstream of his social milieu. In the case of a naturally shy youngster exclusion may create withdrawal which causes him to substantially devalue his personal worth. In turn, feelings of inferiority become all pervasive and influence every aspect of social interaction.

As a group, however, the hearing-impaired listener probably does not experience any greater degrees of frustration than other handicapped subgroups. Because frustration is basically an emotional response to an apparently insoluable conflict, whose alternatives are either unsatisfactory or drastically limited, the handicapped require extraordinary considerations for dealing with their conflicts. Coping mechanisms may take the form of developing increased tolerance to potentially conflicting experiences, seeking compassionate guidance and assistance in dealing with problems or other means. Some psychologists have suggested that frustration serves a useful purpose for stimulating a response of positive action toward finding a sloution to a problem. This reasoning proposes that frustration is simply another motivating force, similar to other basic drives, which can be channeled productively in problem solving.

Hearing Aids -- Anticipation vs. Actuality

To most hearing-impaired individuals the prospect of being fitted with a hearing instrument connotes several different, though related, concepts. Initially, there is the self-realization that only elderly people have to use amplification; ergo, they develop erroneous self-images of maturational levels. Secondly, there is a fear of losing either femininity or masculinity, whatever those concepts mean to their appropriate sex. To a large extent, vanity plays a much greater role in acceptance of amplification than sex-role identification. The hearing aid manufacturers have devoted considerable efforts to achieve a socially-acceptable auditory prosthesis which is both functional as well as cosmetically compatible with "normal" appearance. With the advent within the past several years of in-the-ear instruments there appears to have been greater acceptance of the use of such aids.

Well-established audiologic criteria have generally been adopted for determining the candidacy for amplification by an individual. These include: irreversible sensorineural auditory impairment, whose pure tone average, in the better ear, is 35dB Hearing Level (ANSI 1970) or greater, or exhibits a sensitivity decrease of greater than 45dB Hearing Level at octave frequencies above 1000 Hz; relatively satisfactory word discrimination in quiet and in the presence of moderate background competition. And finally, but perhaps most importantly, the motivation to tolerate certain disadvantages when wearing a hearing instrument, as in high level background acoustical competition, in order to derive the advantages of improved communicative potential under most favorable listening conditions. Of course, for the individual with substantial auditory impairment, there may not exist any reasonable alternative to his communicative difficulty. Thus, he may simply have to tolerate whatever occurs in his acoustical field of experiences.

It is of some significance to members of the hearing health rehabilitation team to realize that many hearing-impaired listeners do not voluntarily seek help for themselves, but rather pursue hearing help at the urging of a spouse or relative. This strongly suggests that the individual refuses to acknowledge the existence of his hearing handicap. Consequently, there is less than total motivation to enter an aural rehabilitation program for the purpose of improving one's own communicative skills. However, family members can and should play a significant role in the supportive end of the rehabilitative process. If at all possible, relatives should be encouraged to adapt their communication skills to the listener's advantage by facing him each time a communicative act occurs, by speaking in turn with others in a group communicative pattern and by speaking in a normal, unexaggerated fashion. Establishing a habitual and advantageous speech pattern can do much to reduce the listener's frustrations and difficulties in everyday functions.

Self Hearing Aid Evaluation

The so-called objective methodology for comparing the electroacoustical-psychoacoustical performance of hearing instruments has fallen into some disrepute within recent years. Because some of the test tools have not carried the high reliability factor which is desirable, many audiologists have simply ceased formal hearing aid evaluations. As a consumer-advocacy stance, however, the hearing aid evaluation procedure might be defended with greater vigor. For the hearing-impaired listener, as a consumer, there is strong governmental support for providing unbiased information which is to the consumer's advantage.

For some hearing-impaired individuals and with the cooperation of ethical hearing aid dispensers, it is possible to perform a self hearing aid evaluation utilizing the old trial-based concepts. This approach permits the prospective hearing aid user to employ an intended instrument under a variety of listening conditions which are more valid than controlled signal-to-noise listening test procedures. In this fashion, the listener can arrive at a realistic conclusion based on his own personal experience which may be a more convincing experience than externally-applied methods. With this form of self-appraisal it is important for the listener to utilize some systematic approach toward his judgements. Thus, his experiences should include those which would be normally experienced everyday during his normal routine of activities. It is helpful to carry a small pad on which can be recorded the time and location of a given listening experience and the subjective reactions of sound quality and comfort of listening. In addition, specific problems of localization of sound, in auditory space, may be noted if deemed important. Also, the conditions under which communication activity occurred should be indicated. For example, was the communication conducted with more than one person, and if so, were there children's and/or women's voices predominant at the time. Over a two week period it should be apparent to the prospective wearer of a hearing instrument whether he can be expected to perform satisfactorily under most conditions, or the specific problems that can occur for adverse situations. In this way, the listener can probably arrive at an intelligent decision regarding the benefits and disadvantages of using personal amplification.

Aural Rehabilitation

A major problem confronting the member of a hearing health team, as well as the client, is the distance and inaccessability readily available for participating in aural rehabilitation activities. Often, the client is elderly and simply cannot obtain satisfactory transportation to the rehabilitation facility for scheduled attendance at training sessions. Perhaps as important a reason for this is the client's perception of passive you-care-for-me-cure model of health care. In other words, the medical model is conceptualized as the only approach to resolving a communication problem. Emphasizing active client participation is an imperative if aural rehabilitation with adults is to succeed. Supportive family involvement is necessary especially with the older client.

The health care professional, obviously, needs to organize his program with definite objectives he hopes to accomplish with any given patient. Initial sessions may be simply oriented toward learning how to operate his new hearing instrument. Subsequently, understanding basic operational concepts of his hearing instrument can be learned. For some individuals, learning how to adjust the gain control of their instruments is a major task and accomplishment allowing them improved discrimination skills. As the hearing-impaired person becomes more adept and skillful in hearing and understanding through auditory training procedures, he can regain confidence in social and other endeavors.

Clearly, the purposes of auditory training are to systematically increase ability to discriminate acoustical stimuli through the exclusive use of the amplifies auditory system. The successof this undertaking, of course, depends upon:
1. nature and magnitude of auditory impairment, ie. pure sensorineural vs. mixed lesions; 2. age and motivation of individual; 3. rewards for efforts expended in training activities. For some listeners, beginning at the primitive level of awareness may be deemed appropriate while others may begin at somewhat more advanced levels of discrimination awareness.

For the child, development of auditory discrimination skills assumes a cooperative and responsive youngster as well as strong support from parents and siblings. Because not all hearing-impaired children receive identical training procedures, nor utilize identical forms of amplification, there exist differences in philosophies and objectives in schools for the deaf and those where children are mainstreamed into regular classrooms. Indeed, Ross (1972) suggests ten "principals" in using amplification in an educational environment. They are: 1. most favorable signal-to-noise ratio, 2. audibility of student's self-vocalizations, 3. communication from student-to-student, 4. early use of amplification, 5. amplify binaurally whenever possible, 6. retain simplicity of electroacoustic transmission system to one type if possible, 7. attenuate sound level as much as possible in the classroom, 8. utilize bisensory (audition and vision) communication, 9. transmission system must be easily maintained, and 10. transmission system must be as flexible as possible.

The employment of hardwire-type transmission systems, as

contrasted to inductance loop amplification (ILA) and radio frequency transmission systems (RF), leave a great deal to be desired. The hardwire system, because it utilizes connecting wires, obviously restricts the physical activities and range of motion of the youngster. Moreover, its presence, in some respects, can almost be considered hazardous to tripping and walking in the classroom. On the other hand, the wireless type systems permit greater physical flexibility for teacher and child within the classroom and outdoors and still manage to maintain auditory contact and communication. The disadvantage to the youngster lies in the fact that many programs do not allow the child to utilize the same receiver unit in his out-of-school setting activities. Consequently, the child very often must try to learn to discriminate sounds utilizing two differing sets of acoustic signals which probably contain disparate acoustic clues for identification. Clearly, if the purpose of auditory training is to increase the auditory perceptual skills of the listener, then a consistent, reliable system of amplification should form the basis of the entire process. Otherwise, much of what we can hope to be accomplished will be left up to chance occurrence.

The adult with auditory impairment experiences a less than global form of perceptual difficulty with acoustical information. Instead, he has a well-developed language and communication system and has been functioning at a social symbolic level of activity. More often than not, the main difficulty lies in speech-sound patterns of discrimination. In general, there tends to be need to regain basic speech phoneme identification, which, for some listeners, is a monumental achievement. Because this may not always be possible, many moderately-severe hearing impaired individuals must supplement auditory clues with speech (lip) reading information. The combination of bisensory inputs usually can provide the additional communicative clues required to achieve a satisfactory communicative exchange.

Multiple Handicaps

The coexistence of several handicapping conditions of course makes it more difficult for the individual to manage and cope with his communication difficulty. The deaf-blind, clearly, require training and considerations from an individual with a high degree of training and specialization beyond the scope of this discussion. The degree to which other non-communicative impairments affect the individual's well being must reflect an extension of his adjustment to his overall difficulties in social intercourse. Should the other conditions constitute major problems in social-vocational areas, then team-type efforts most certainly are indicated. Many disciplines, including psychology, social work, physical and occupational therapies and rehabilitation counseling need to be brought into the situation.

Among some of the problems which the hearing-impaired person experiences is tinnitus or head noises in one or both ears. Tinnitus has been documented to occur in both the normal as well as hearing-impaired populations. However, a large segment of the sensorineurally-impaired population represent transistory or constant tinnitus to a substantial degree for whom little help has been available. Although some early studies of tinnitus suggested neurotic-leaning personalities, clinical experience has tended to suggest that there is no greater neurotic tendency among tinnitus sufferers than among the general non-impaired population as a whole. Whatever the etiologies of tinnitus may be, it is probable that the experience can serve as a focal point symptom toward which any anxiety-prone individual can conveniently point a finger. The history of medical treatment of tinnitus has ranged from surgical section of the 8th cranial nerve to a spectrum of medications to acupuncture to biofeedback. None of these forms of treatment have proven to be satisfactory for the alleviation of the condition. Recently, however, a tinnitus study and treatment group headed by Vernon at the University of Oregon School of Health Sciences, has reported a moderate degree of success in relieving the sympton utilizing a tinnitus masking approach. While this approach does appear to show promise for some tinnitus-hearing-impaired individuals, only continued study will be able to verify its long-term benefits.

The presence of vertigo or true dizziness, as contrasted to lightheadedness, often accompanies some forms of hearing impairment, particularly the end organ disease of Meniere's Syndrome. The basis of this disorder may reside at the peripheral vestibular-controlling mechanism, semicircular canals, or at a more "central" anatomical location, either of which can only be discerned by electronystagmography. In contrast to tinnitus, vertigo, particularly of the peripherally-based type, can be medically managed fairly successfully. It must be remembered. however, that vertigo is an extremely distressing symptom with potentially debilitating and depressing consequences for many individuals.

Management of Aural Rehabilitation

The initial or short period of acclimation to the acceptance and/or rejection of personal amplification for some hearing-impaired persons becomes evident within a one week period. That this is a distinctly unsatisfactory experience or prospect can often be discerned at the time of fitting. Certain personality characteristics or attitudes are often manifested which verbally are not simply doubtful, but are usually totally negative. An example is, "I know Aunt Lilly tried one once and it never helped her, so I know it won't help me". Or, "I know I'll bring it back in a week". Clearly in such situations, the hearing health team member must first gain the patient's confidence before it is possible to proceed with any aspect of aural rehabilitation procedures. In general, it is most important to have a supportive family member along with the patient, someone who can render positive reinforcement and intelligent understanding of the situation.

For the early adjustment period there are two time-controlled criteria that have been helpful for acceptance of personal amplification: one is the gradual usage of the instrument in increased hours of wearing same. The other delimits the listening situations to those which are, to begin with, most familiar to the patient, ie., home, outdoor neighbor contact and so forth. Irregardless of which criterion is selected as the guiding principle, there is need for strong and positive suppotive statements from all concerned. Such an approach must be integrated with realistic expectations of what amplification can and cannot accomplish as discussed earlier.

Over the long term, the management of the aided hearing-impaired listener requires periodic checks for any number of reasons. Obviously, if there is a persistence of chronic otopathology, that requires medical management for its control. The clinician or hearing health team member concerned with the instrument needs to assure proper mechanical function of the hearing aid. Thus, periodic cleaning should be accomplished at least once or twice yearly and repairs performed as necessary for proper gain, output and switching functions. This can become a major problem in geographic areas where salt air is prevalent. Use of desiccants and other self-help cleaning of earmolds should be conveyed to the patient as routine aspects of instrument care. It is vital to the hearing-impaired listener, wearing amplification, that he receive the benefit of long tern attention and necessary support. As a final comment on long-term management, it is suggested that the clinician, like the physician, make himself available over the long term and in emergencies where substitute amplification may need to be made available.

Summary

Auditory impairment can precipitate a multitude of problems all of which are essentially centered around communicative skills difficulties. The ramifications of hearing loss extend well beyond the immediate family ties and include virtually all avenues of psychosocial interactions. The hearing health professional, if he is to render a truly important function, must learn to understand the problems which confront the individual in his daily life. In order to effectively deal with, and provide the support necessary for rehabilitation, the clinician must understand that some personality concepts are often altered to the detriment of the individual. It is well known, for example, that certain responses are elicited when the hearing-impaired listener is confronted with his difficulties and is under pressures to cope with society. An initial reaction is denial, which in a more extreme form is an obliteration of personal involvement with others and hearing. Secondly, projection can occur, which is employed to cast the responsibility of his inabilities onto others. Thirdly, withdrawal from social and other forms of interactions diminishes the need for responsible communication skills, and lastly, permanent alteration of self-image.

The primary objective of aural rehabilitaion, of course, is to restore communication skills to their original or as closely as possible, pre-impairment level. Almost invariably, an important component of this process will involve the utilization of personal amplification. It is vitally important that realistic expectations be understood by the auditorially-handicapped person. That is, there are advantages as well as disadvantages to the use of amplification. Under certain conditions, particularly quiet listening, discrimination performance should substantially improve. On the other hand, under varying levels of noise, discrimination abilities will be affected adversely. Acceptance of these facts are important to long-term successful usage of amplification.

Short-term management should strive to involved frequent and periodic contact with the patient. Involvement should revolve around communicative situations where great difficulty is encountered and usage of amplification may be advantageously employed. As before, continued positive reinforcement and support to the individual is imperative, particularly if this can be achieved through nuclear family involvement.

The presence of multiple or coexisting problems such as tinnitus, vertigo, or other physical limitations, increases the coping task of the hearing-impaired. Dealing with unresolved vertigo may simply be too devastating when combined with hearing loss. Thus, medical management of vertigo is imperative and should be controlled prior to other management. At this stage, it may be necessary to bring several disciplines into the patient's management arena and that should be achieved as quickly as possible.

In summary, pre- and post-fitting counseling are imperatives which cannot be left to chance, but must be planned intelligently.

References

American National Standards Specifications for Audiometers, New York, Amer. Nat. Stds. Inst., (1970).

Bender, L., Contributions to Developmental Neuropsychiatry, New York, International University Press, (1964).

Ross, M., Principles of Aural Rehabilitation, New York, Bobbs-Merrill, (1972).

Schilder, P., Contributions to Developmental Neuropsychiatry, New York, International University Press, (1964).

Wright, B., Physical Disability, A Psychological Approach, New Jersey, Prentice-Hall, (1955).

Chapter 10

Audibility and Intelligibility of Speech for Listeners with Sensorineural Hearing Loss

Margaret W. Skinner, Ph.D.

The purpose of this paper is 1) to describe a method for comparing a statistical value of the speech spectrum with the dynamic range of a hard-of-hearing listener, and 2) to explain how this method has been coupled with a parametric approach for estimating the optimum frequency-response and overall-gain characteristics of a hearing aid.

I. Method for comparing a statistical value of the speech spectrum with the dynamic range of a hard-of-hearing listener.

The accurate comparison of the listener's dynamic range with a statistical value of the speech spectrum is dependent on both stimuli being measured at the same point of reference. In this paper the point of reference was the approximate center of the listener's head, unless otherwise noted, and the stimuli were third-octave bands of noise and the words from the Pascoe High-Frequency Word List (Pascoe, 1975). These measurements are shown for one listener in Figure 1. The third-octave bands of noise, with which the thresholds of audibility and disconfort were determined, were measured on the slow, RMS scale. The thresholds of audibility were obtained with a clinical method of limits, with a 1-dB stepsize near threshold. The thresholds of discomfort were obtained with a method of adjustment according to the following criterion: the intensity level 1-dB below which the listener would not like to listen for long time. The word levels were determined in the following manner. Each word of the Pascoe High Fre-

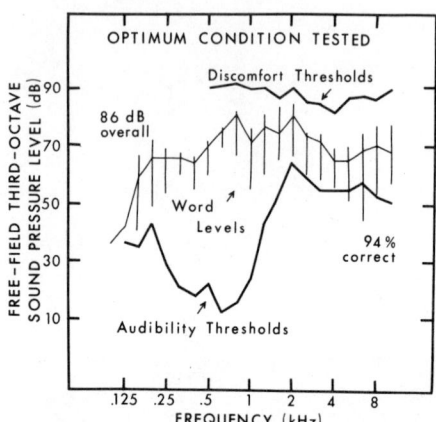

Figure 1. Comparison of a listener's dynamic range with a statistical value of the speech spectrum. The listener's thresholds of audibility and discomfort were obtained with third octave bands of noise centered at the stated frequencies. The word-level contour represents the 75th percentile of the third octave SPL of the words of the Pascoe High-Frequency Word List The vertical, thin lines represent the 10th to 90th percentile range of these measurements. The overall intensity level, which is the mean of the intensity levels for the 50 words measured on the RMS-slow linear scale, is shown at the left of the word-level contour. The listener's word-identification score for this frequency-response and overall gain condition is shown at the right of the figure. The sound-level measurements and testing were done in a free-field.

quency Word List was captured in a one-second integrating window and the equivalent root-mean-squared (RMS) sound pressure level (SPL: re 20 µPa), in each third-octave band was obtained (see Skinner, 1976 for procedure) for each of twenty-one bands. This resulted in 50 measurements for each of the one third-octave bands for this frequency response and overall intensity level. The 75th percentile of this distribution of measures (that is, the levels exceeded 25% of the time) was calculated for each of the third-octave bands and is represented by the thin-lined contour in Figure 1. The 75th percentile was chosen instead of the 50th because at least 250 milliseconds (msec) of silence was included in the integrating window. The range from the 90th to the 10th percentile level of the words is represented by the vertical, thin lines. In addition, the overall intensity level of each word was measured with a sound level meter set to the RMS-slow-linear re-

sponse, The average of these numbers, shown at the left of
the word-level contour, is 86 dB SPL. The word-identification
score in percent correct is shown at the right of the figure.

When the data are displayed in this manner, one can visually compare the intensity level of the speech energy in
each band with the listener's dynamic range. From this data
one can give approximate answers to the following questions.
Is the speech energy audible, and if so, where is it within
the dynamic range? Does it exceed the listener's threshold
of discomfort at any band? How does the listener's score relate to the configuration and overall intensity level of the
word-level contour? Answers to these questions are important
bases for our choice of parameters to test in our search for
the optimum frequency-response and gain characteristics of
amplification for the individual listener.

II. Application of this comparison of word-levels and dynamic range to optimizing frequency-response and gain
characteristics.

A. Skinner investigation.

This investigation (Skinner, 1976; 1979) was with six
listeners with noise-induced hearing losses. Their pure tone
audiograms (air conduction) for the test ear are shown in
Figure 2. From 125 through 1000 Hz their thresholds are within normal limits; at 2000 Hz their thresholds were equal to
or greater than 45 dB Hearing Threshold Level (HTL). None
had a conductive hearing loss, and all had complete recruitment (Alternate Binaural Loudness Balance Test; Fowler, 1950)

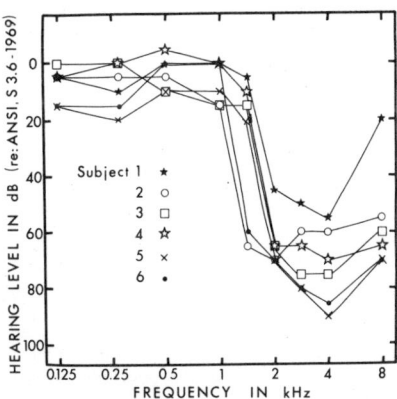

Figure 2. Pure tone, air conduction thresholds for the test
esr of the six listeners in the Skinner investigation.

and positive Short Increment Sensitivity Index scores at 20 dB sensation level (SL) (Jerger, Shedd and Harford, 1959) at 200 Hz.

The research design was as follows. For Experiment I, five frequency responses were chosen in an attempt to bracket the region in which the best one lay. Frequency Response I was a nominally uniform response, and Frequency Responses II through V were designed to compensate for the high-frequency hearing loss of the listeners. There was 0-dB compensation from 100 through 500 Hz, and increasing amounts of high-frequency emphasis (in 11-dB steps) from 1600 to 10,000 Hz. The amount of emphasis between 500 and 1600 Hz was defined by the low-frequency boundary of each listener's hearing loss. The Pascoe High-Frequency Word List spoken by a female talker was amplified with the system set for each of these frequency responses, and at five levels of overall intensity from soft to very loud. In Experiment II, the frequency response associated with the highest scores in Experiment I was modified in an attempt tp approximate the optimum response more closely. The sequence of conditions for both experiments was counterbalanced to distribute learning and fatigue effects.

Unlike other investigations of compensatory amplification, the high-frequency emphasis preceded the loudspeaker. That is, the processing which usually occurs in a master hearing aid or wearable aid was included in the speech-amplification circuit. In this situation, the uniform response defined the "unaided condition", and functional or real-ear gain for the "aided conditions" was determined by calculating the difference in dB between the compensatory frequency response and the uniform response for each third-octave band between 100 and 10,000 Hz. The amplification system was linear, that is, there was no output limiting or compression, and the distortion was not significant even at the highest intensity levels tested.

To explore the relation between the 75th percentile levels of the words and the dynamic range of the listeners, word-level contours were plotted for each frequency response and overall intensity level employed in Experiment I. When the data are presented in this way, there appears to be at least three factors that affect the word-identification score for a single frequency response and intensity level. These are: 1) how much of the spectrum of a word exceeds the listener's threshold, that is, the audibility of the acoustic energy in each band, 2) the balance between the level in a high-frequency band between 2 and 4 KHz and the level in a low-frequency band between 500 and 1000 Hz, and 3) the separation of the band levels of the words from the threshold of discomfort. Audibility is clearly the most important of these three factors.

The audibility of the speech energy in individual bands can be deduced from a comparison of the 75th percentile levels with the audibility threshold for the appropriate band. For example, look at the graphs for Frequency Responses III and IV for Listener 2 in Figure 3. Large increments in score

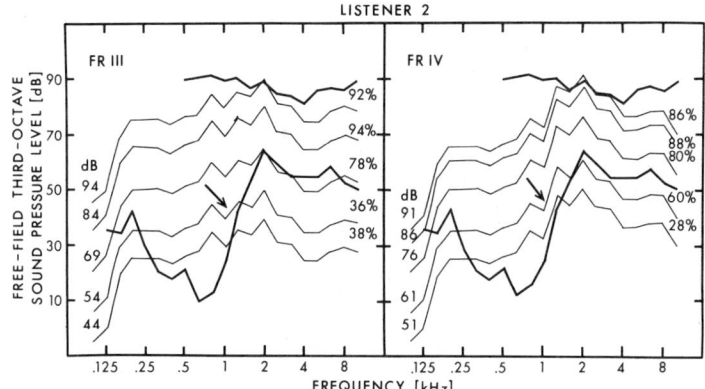

Figure 3. Comparison of the word-level contours for Frequency Responses III and IV with Listener 2's dynamic range. The overall intensity level of the word-list is at the left of the word level contours, and the word-identification score is at the right. The arrows point to the mid-frequency region which is inaudible for Frequency Response III and audible for Frequency Response IV. (See caption for Fig. 1 for a more complete description of the stimuli.)

were associated with increases in the sensation level (SL) of the low-frequency bands of the words. In addition, a significant increase in score was associated with audibility of the speech energy at 1.6 and 2 KHz. Compare the word-level contours for the overall intensity levels of 54 and 61 dB SPL for Frequency Responses III and IV respectively. In Frequency Response III the speech energy at 1.6 and 2 KHz was inaudible, whereas with Frequency Response IV, this energy was audible. There was a 24% increase in score associated with audibility of this mid-frequency energy. Similar increments in score occurred for the other listeners.

The importance of the appropriate balance between the low- and high-frequency speech energy is reflected in the scores of Listener 2, as shown in Figure 4. The word levels associated with the uniform response (FR I) are shown in the top graph, those with 22-dB high-frequency emphasis (FR III) in the middle graph, and those with 44-dB emphasis (FR V) in the bottom graph. It is evident that too much high-frequency

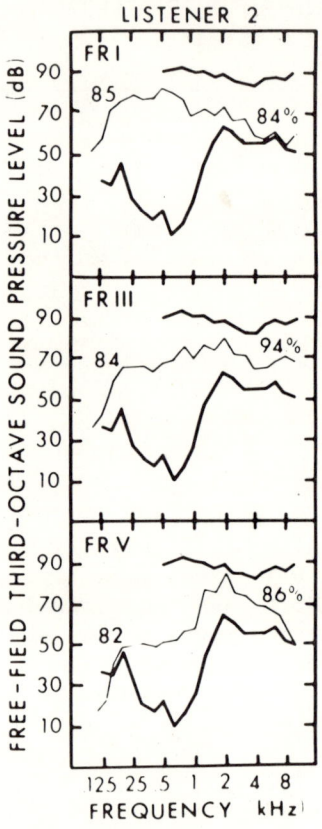

Figure 4. Comparison of word-level contours for Frequency Responses I, III, and V with Listener 2's dynamic range. The word-identification score associated with Frequency Response III is significantly higher than for the other two responses, despite the fact that the overall level was approximately the same, and the speech energy was audible for all three.

emphasis, or none at all, is associated with significantly lower scores than when there is the appropriate amount of emphasis, even when the overall level is approximately the same and the speech energy is within the listener's dynamic range. (In this study a 5% difference in score was statistically significant at the 0.05 level of confidence.) The scores associated with the word-level contours in this figure were higher than for any other overall level tested for the respective frequency response.

When the band levels of the words reached or surpassed the discomfort level, the scores decreased. This adverse effect of surpassing the discomfort level is shown clearly in Frequency Response II for Listener 4 in Figure 5. When the

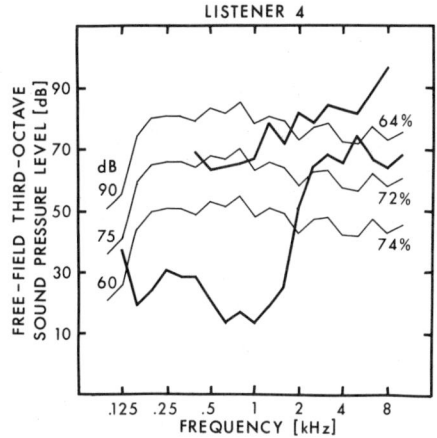

Figure 5. Comparison of three word-level contours for Frequency Response II for Listener 4 with his dynamic range. His word-identification score was significantly higher for an overall intensity level of 60 dB SPL than it was for 90 dB SPL. With the 90-dB condition of the speech energy below 1600 Hz surpassed his thresholds of discomfort.

words were presented at an overall level of 90 dB SPL, this listener's score of 64% was significantly less (10%) than when the words were presented at 60 dB SPL. Listeners 1, 2, 5 and 6 also showed this same decrease in performance as some band levels of the words exceeded the threshold of discomfort.

The word-level contours associated with the highest word-identification score for each listener from both experiments are shown in Figure 6. The frequency response and gain characteristics associated with these word-level contours approximate the optimum since they were intermediate among the conditions tested. There are two important observations which can be made about these contours. The first observation concerns their position within the listener's dynamic range. For all listeners the 75th percentile levels of the words ex-

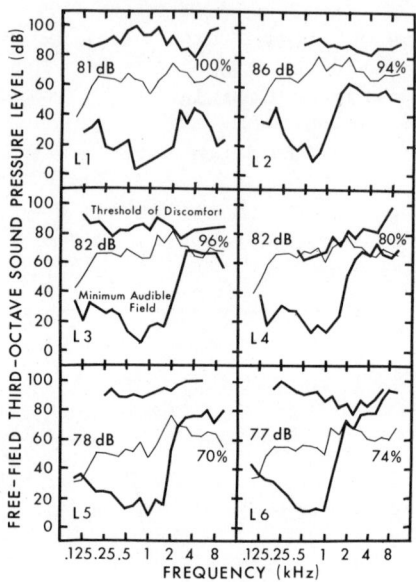

Figure 6. Comparison of the word-level contour, associated with the highest word-identification score, with the dynamic range of the six listeners in the Skinner investigation. The overall intensity level is shown at the left of the word-level contour and the word-identification score at the right. These represent the optimum condition tested for each listener.

ceed the thresholds of audibility for all listeners through 2 KHz, and for those listeners with less loss, they are audible to 10 KHz. Although most-comfortable-loudness (MCL) judgements for third-octave bands of noise were not obtained, the word levels at 1 KHz and below (except for Listeners 5 and 6) are within the range of MCL for a group of normally hearing listeners (Mantovani, Pascoe and Skinner, 1978). For the hearing-impaired listeners it was particularly important to have the word levels between 1.25 and 2 KHz at a positive sensation level (SL); when energy was eliminated in this region in Experiment II there was a significant decrement in scores. Furthermore, the word levels did not exceed the threshold of discomfort except for Listener 4 whose criterion was unusually strict. These results, obtained with linear amplification, suggest that the words need to be amplified so that their energy falls within the listener's dynamic range for maximum intelligibility.

A second observation is that maximum intelligibility was associated with a narrow range of overall output levels (77 to 86 dB SPL) despite the individual differences in high-frequency emphasis needed tp compensate for the hearing loss. To achieve these optimum levels, the listeners with less loss (Listeners 1 through 4) needed 10 to 15 dB more overall gain and less high-frequency emphasis than those with greater losses (Listeners 5 and 6). This trade-off in the amount of energy in different spectral regions to achieve the same overall output is reminiscent of the concern of the Committee on Electro-acoustics (1947) with the balance between amplification bandwidth and overall power. These results suggest that we need to explore further the high- and low-frequency cut-offs which are associated with maximum intelligibility.

The frequency responses, which were associated with the highest word-identification scores in the Skinner study, are shown in Figure 7. These responses, which are expressed in

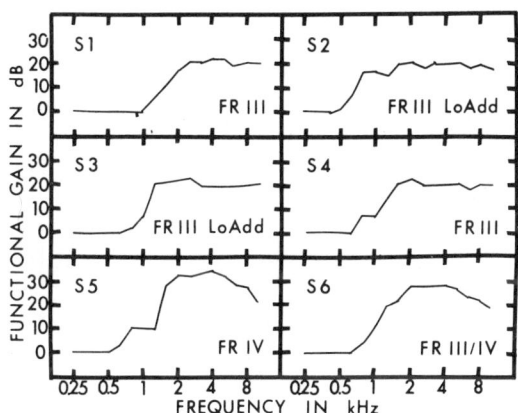

Figure 7. The frequency responses associated with the optimum condition tested for each of the six listeners in the Skinner investigation. See the text for the procedure by which the functional gain was obtained.

terms of functional or real-ear gain, are the same ones which produced the speech spectra in Figure 6. The amount of high-frequency emphasis between 2 and 10 KHz varied from 20 to 33 dB, when there was 0 dB gain from 100 to 500 Hz. The functional gain between 500 and 1600 Hz represented the difference between the listener's audibility curve and the normal curve. These results closely resemble those of Lippman (1978) and Barfod et al. (1971) (if the latter results are converted to real-ear gain) for listeners with similar high-frequency hearing losses. The amount of high-frequency emphasis is approximately 10 dB more than Pascoe (1975) found was best for a group of eight listeners with gently sloping, sensorineural hearing losses.

B. Mantovani, Skinner and Pascoe investigation (1978)

The purpose of this investigation was to apply several strategies for optimizing the frequency response and gain characteristics of amplification fro two listeners with sharply sloping hearing losses. Their audiograms for the test ear are shown in Figure 8. Note that their hearing losses begin

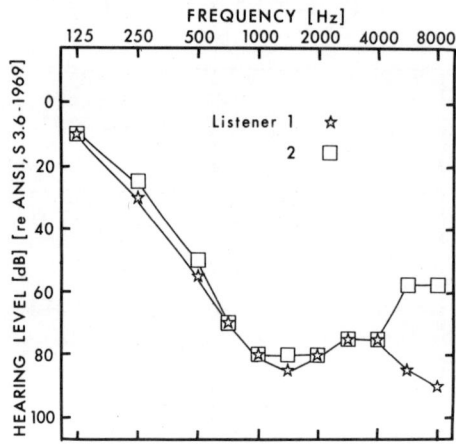

Figure 8. Pure-tone, air-conduction thresholds for the two listeners in the Mantovani, Skinner and Pascoe (1978) investigation

at about 250 Hz and are severe in the high frequencies. Neither of them has a conductive hearing loss. The strategy for determining the emphasis given to the uniform response in each third-octave band was as follows. Each listener's thresholds of audibility and discomfort as well as their MCL[1] judgments for third-octave bands of noise were plotted (see Figure 9). In addition, Pascoe's (1978) "perceived spectra of

---

[1] The criterion for MCL was the level which would be most comfortable to listen to over a long period of time. The method of adjustment was used to obtain the MCL.

summed speech" were plotted to represent mean average speech levels (see contour B in both graphs in Figure 9) for an overall level of 65 dB SPL. Contour A represents the intensity levels to which we wanted contour B amplified. The vertical lines with arrows represent the difference in dB between these two contours for each third-octave band.

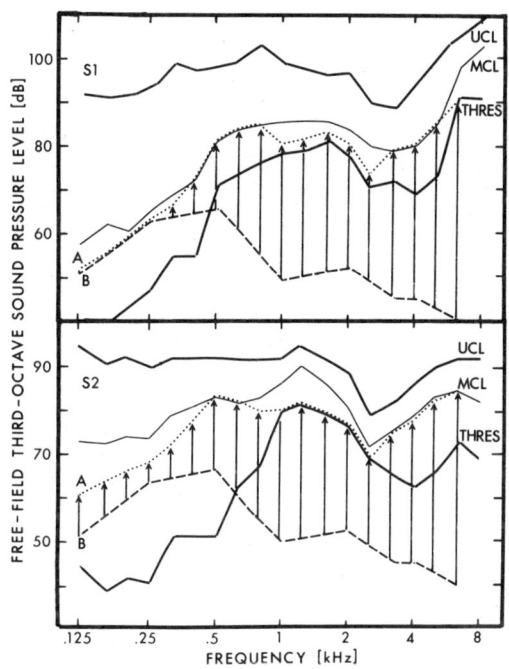

Figure 9. Strategy by which the reference frequency response was chosen for each of the two listeners for Experiment I. The thresholds of audibility and discomfort, as well as MCL, were obtained with third-octave bands of noise centered at the stated frequencies. Contour A represents the intensity level to which we wanted to amplify the "perceived spectra of summed speech" (Pascoe, 1978), which is represented by Contour B. The vertical arrows represent the gain in dB at each third-octave band which was added to the uniform response. The sound-level measurements were made with third-octave-band analysis in the free-field.

The Pascoe High-Frequency Word List spoken by male talker was amplified with the system set for 1) the above reference

frequency response, 2) two degrees of less emphasis in the
high frequencies, and 3) a nominally uniform response. The
amplification system employed for the Skinner investigation
was also used for this study. That is, it was a linear system in which processing occurred in the speech-amplification
circuit and not in a master hearing aid. The listeners adjusted the overall level of the words to MCL with the system
set for each of the frequency-response conditions. The word
lists were presented at MCL for all of the responses and at
+6 dB MCL for the compensatory frequency responses. The sequence of conditions was counterbalanced to distribute the
effects of learning and fatigue. For comparison, each listener adjusted the gain of a wearable hearing aid to MCL for
the words amplified with the system set for the uniform response and an overall gain of 65 dB SPL.

The word levels for the Pascoe High-Frequency Word List,
measured according to the procedure described earlier, are
shown in relation to Listener 1's dynamic range in Figure 10.

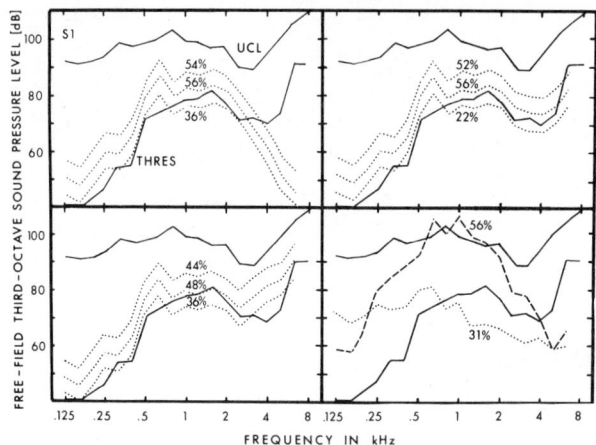

Figure 10. Comparison of the word-level contours, derived
from measurements of the Pascoe High-Frequency Word List spoken by a male talker, with Listener 1's dynamic range. The
reference frequency response, which was chosen by the strategy depicted in Figure 9, was employed for obtaining the results shown in the lower, left-hand block. Two degrees of
high-frequency de-emphasis of this reference response were
employed for obtaining the results shown in the upper two
blocks. The middle, word-level contour of these three blocks
was associated with the overall level chosen as MCL. The dotted-line contour in the lower, right-hand block represents
the word levels measured with the amplification system set

Fig. 10 con't. - for the uniform response and MCL. The dashed line represents the word-level contour derived for the words amplified 1)with the system set for the uniform response for 65 dB SPL overall, and 2) with his own wearable hearing aid set at MCL for this signal level. The word-identification contour is also shown.

The results for the reference frequency response are shown in the lower, left-hand block. Notice that the maximum score of 48% is significantly less tahn the scores obtained with less high-frequency emphasis as shown in the upper two blocks. Also note the small decrement in score when the words were amplified at 6 dB above MCL for each of the compensatory frequency responses. The dotted line in the lower, right-hand block represents the word-level contour for the uniform response adjusted to MCL. When the system was set at MCL for the best compensatory responses, his score was 25% higher than with the uniform response. This difference in score appears to be the result of two interrelated factors: 1) the balance between the spectral energy in the low- and high-frequency regions, and 2) the audibility of the spectral energy above 630 Hz. With the uniform response the overall intensity level reached MCL before the spectral energy above 630 Hz became audible, whereas with the compensatory response there was less low-frequency energy and the high-frequency energy was audible for an overall intensity which was confortably loud. These results indicate the importance of frequency-selective amplification for maximizing speech intelligibility.

Listener 1, who has worn his hearing aid for a number of years, has learned to identify many of the acoustic cues of speech with the amplification which it provides. His score with this aid was identical to his maximum score with the laboratory system, despite the fact that the word-levels exceeded his threshold of discomfort between 630 and 1600 Hz (see the dashed line in the lower, right-hand block of Figure 10). These "aided" word levels were not measured but calculated in the following manner. The functional gain of his hearing aid, set at the gain employed for testing, was calculated by subtracting his aided from his unaided thresholds for third-octave bands of noise. This functional gain at each third-octave band was then added to the word levels measured with the system set for the uniform response and an overall intensity level of 65 dB SPL. It is possible that with a period of training this listener would get a higher score with the laboratory system (if it were made into a wearable aid) than with his own hearing aid.

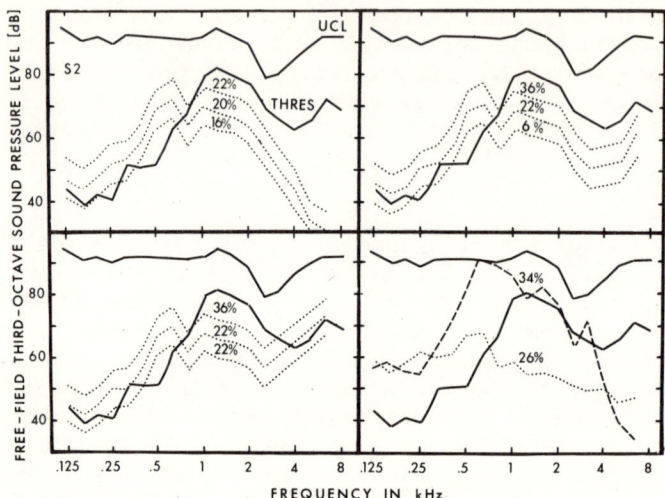

Figure 11. Comparison of the word-level contours, derived from measurements of the Pascoe High-Frequency Word List spoken by a male talker, with Listener 2's dynamic range. The reference frequency response, which was chosen by the strategy depicted in Fig. 9, was employed for obtaining the results shown in the lower, left-hand block. Two degrees of high-frequency de-emphasis of this reference response were employed for obtaining the results shown in the upper two blocks. The middle, word-level contour of these three blocks was associated with the overall level chosen as MCL. The dotted line contour in the lower, right-hand block represents the word-levels measured with the amplification system set for the uniform responses and MCL. The dashed line represents the word-level contour derived for the words amplified 1) with the system set for the uniform response for 65 dB SPL overall, and 2) with a wearable hearing aid set at MCL for this signal level. The word-identification score associated with each word-level contour is also shown.

The results for Listener 2 are shown in Figure 11. This listener has worn a hearing aid only for a few periods of several hours, because she has found the loud sound very irritating. It is significant that, when she set the overall output of the laboratory system to her MCL, the words were only audible between 250 and 630 Hz, a situation which approximates her hearing of speech in everyday life. Her highest scores (36%) are associated with the highest word-level contours, shown in the upper, right-hand block and the lower, left-hand block. The major difference between these two contours and the highest word-level contour in the upper, left-hand block is the amount of energy between 2.5 and 6.3 KHz. Although it appears that this energy is below the threshold of audibility for the contour in the upper, right-hand block, apparently it is contributing to the 14% higher score than was obtained with the condition represented by the highest contour in the upper, left-hand block. It appears that the particular RMS measurement of the word levels employed in this study is underestimating, especially in the high-frequency range, the energy which must be audible. It is probable that a measurement of the 10% cumulative levels, such as has been made by Lippman (1978) and Barfod (1976), would be more appropriate. Listener 2's score with a wearable hearing aid (borrowed from our clinic) set to MCL was approximately the same as with the laboratory system. With the system set for the uniform response and for the overall level of the words at MCL, her score was 10% worse than with the best compensatory response. These results again support the need for frequency-selective amplification.

In a second experiment with these two listeners, we changed our strategy for setting the reference frequency response. As shown in Figure 12, we added about 5 and 18 dB emphasis between 200 and 630 Hz, and 6 dB more at 2.5 KHz for Listener 1. The low-frequency emphasis caused the mean average speech levels between 200 and 400 Hz substantially higher than this listener's MCL for third-octave bands of noise. The reference frequency response for Listener 2 was determined empirically by adjusting channel gain so that she could discriminate between the phonemes /s/ and /ʃ/. Consequently, we gave far less emphasis at all frequency bands except 2 and 2.5 KHz, and the gain in bands centered at 1 and 1.25 KHz was turned all the way down. The choice of modifications of the reference frequency response was different for the two listeners. For Listener 1 we paired three settings of the high-frequency (4 through 6.3 KHz) channel gain with three settings of the low-frequency (200 through 400 Hz) channel gain. In addition, we employed one frequency response with a central notch. For Listener 2, we chose five high-frequency cut-offs (2.5 through 5 KHz) and three low-frequency modifications (between 200 and 400 Hz) of the reference frequency response. In addition, we employed one frequency response without the notch.

The results for both listeners indicate that there is an optimum bandwidth which is less than that of the reference frequency response (200 through 6300 Hz). The results for

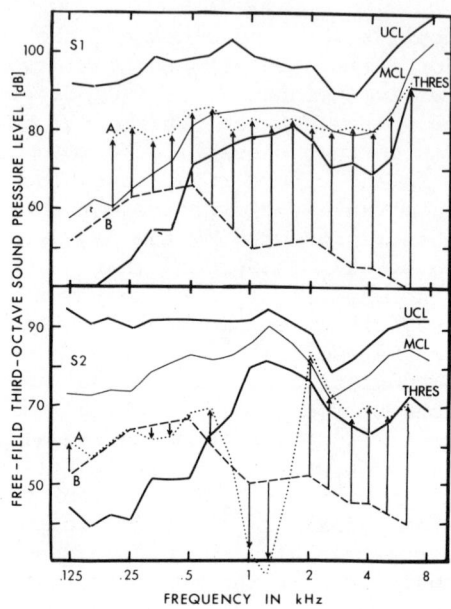

Figure 12. Strategy by which the reference frequency response was chosen for each of the two listeners for Experiment II. The thresholds of audibility and discomfort as well as MCL were obtained with third-octave bands of noise centered at the stated frequencies. Contour A represents the intensity level to which we wanted to amplify the "perceived spectra of summed speech" (Pascoe, 1978), which is represented by Contour B. The vertical arrows represent the gain in dB at each third-octave band which was added to the uniform response. Note that there was negative gain for several bands for Listener 2. The sound level measurements were made with third-octave band analysis in a free-field.

Listener 1 are shown in Figure 13. The highest score (60%) is associated with a frequency response with cut-offs below 300 Hz and above 4000[2] Hz (see the two, left-hand blocks); however, frequency responses with low- and high-frequency cut-

---

[2] The actual bandwidth at the 3-dB down points was 282 to 4470 Hz. The values 300 Hz and 4000 Hz represent the center frequencies of the lowest and highest bands. Subsequent unpublished research with output limiting at the threshold of discomfort for this listener suggests that his highest performance is associated with an actual bandwidth from 266 to 6 KHz.

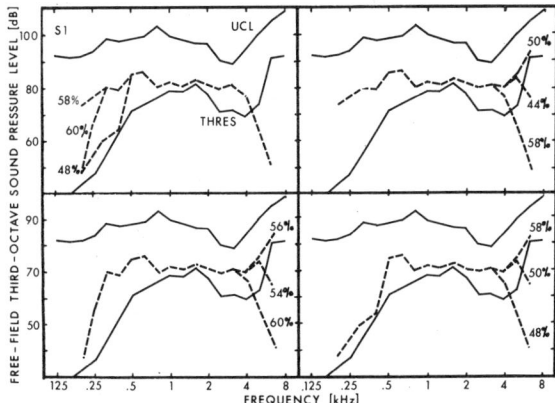

Figure 13. Comparison of the word-level contours associated with the reference frequency response and its modifications with the dynamic range of Listener 1 for Experiment II. In the upper, left-hand block are plotted the word-level contours associated with the low-frequency modifications and one high-frequency modification. In the upper, right-hand block are plotted the word-level contours associated with the reference frequebcy response and two high-frequency modifications of it. In the lower two blocks are plotted the word-level contours associated with the three high-frequency settings of the frequency response and two degrees of low-frequency de-emphasis. The word-identification score associated with each word-level contour is also shown.

offs of 200 and 4000 Hz (see the upper left-hand block, contour associated with 58%), 300 and 6300 Hz (see the lower, left-hand block, contour associated with 56%), and 500 and 6300 Hz (see the lower, right-hand block, contour associated with 58%) respectively are associated with scores that are not significantly lower. These results support the observation made of the Skinner data that there appears to be an optimum overall intensity level which is associated with maximum intelligibility.

The results for the two listeners with the amplification system set for the mid-frequency notch (at 1 and 1.25 KHz) were not significantly different from those without the notch (see Figure 14). For Listener 1, the score was slightly improved by putting in the notch, but this may have occurred because the overall level was lower. For Listener 2, the score was slightly higher with no notch. However, it is possible that the use of the notch would have resulted in slightly

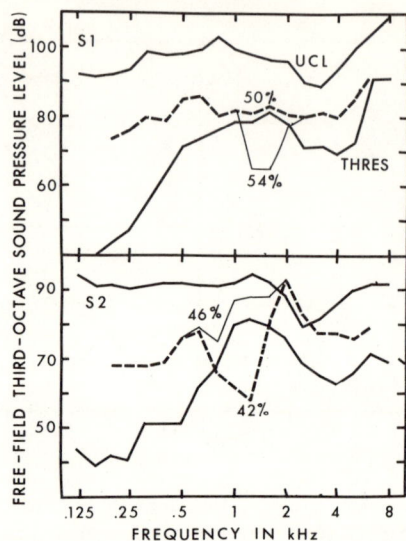

Figure 14. Comparison of the word-level contours for the reference frequency response (dashed line) and its mid-frequency modification (thin line) with the dynamic range of the two listeners. The word-identification score associated with the word-level contours is also shown.

higher scores had there been more energy in the low frequencies.

The results for Listener 2 for the various low- and high- frequency modifications of the reference frequency respone are shown in Figure 15. This reference frequency responce gave no gain to the average speech levels from 200 to 500 Hz which meant that the speech energy was at least 10 dB below MCL in this region. Further decreases of the energy in this region were associated with significant decrements in score. These scores were 10 to 20% less than without this decrease in low-frequency energy. The scores associated with the high-frequency modification seem to indicate that energy above approximately 5000 Hz is not necessary for maximum intelligibility, but that decreases at 4000 Hz and below were associated with significantly lower scores.

In summary, the results from these two experiments employing linear amplification seem to support the hypothesis that maximum speech intelligibility for these listeners with sensorineural hearing loss is associated with an optimum overall intensity level. Furthermore, there is ample evidence that frequency-selective amplification is necessary to shape the spectral energy so that it is audible throughout

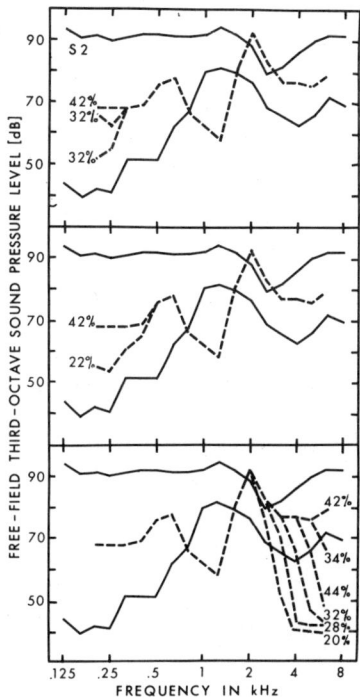

Figure 15. Comparison of the word-level contours, associated with the reference frequency response and its modifications, with the dynamic range for Listener 2 for Experiment II. In the upper two blocks are shown the word-level contours associated with the reference frequency response and low-frequency modifications of it. In the lowest block is shown the word-level contours associated with the reference frequency response and its high-frequency modifications. The word-identification score associated with each word-level contour is also shown.

the amplified frequency range. It is only with this shaping that speech intelligibility can be maximized for this optimum overall intensity level.

C. Limiting Master Hearing Aid.

Since our work with linear amplification indicated that speech needs to be spectrally shaped and output limited to maximize intelligibility, a limiting master hearing aid was designed and built at Central Institute for the Deaf (Barth,

Heidbreder, Niemoeller, Miller and Skinner, 1977) to fulfill both of these functions. A schematic diagram of this hearing aid is shown in Figure 16. With this aid the spectrum is di-

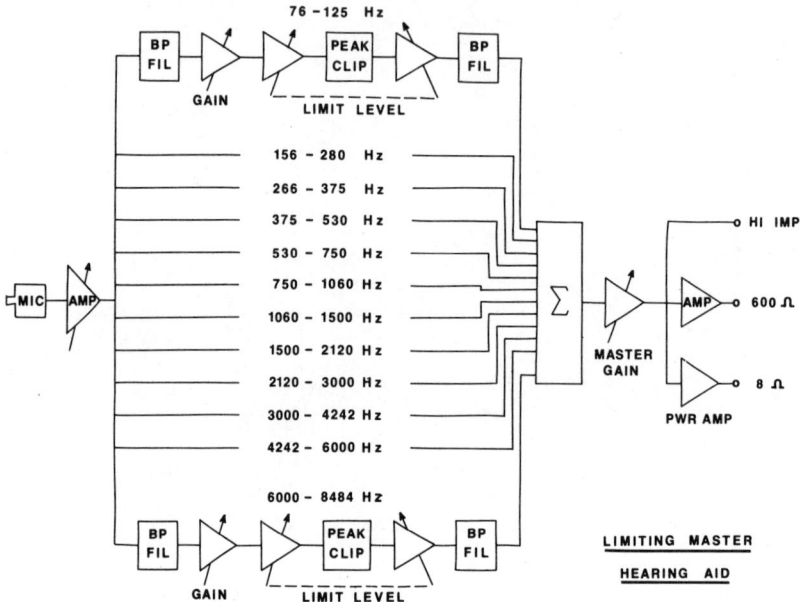

Figure 16. A block diagram of the limiter master hearing aid.

vided into 12 channels by a bank of band-pass filters, ten of which are spaced at one half-octave intervals (center frequencies from 322 through 7242 Hz) and have bandwidths of one-half octave. The lowest two channels (centered at 100 and 211 Hz) are approximately an octave apart with bandwidths of about 0.8 octave. The gain in each channel is controlled by an amplifier, and the limit is established by appropriately ganging an amplifier, a nonlinear element and a second amplifier. The two amplifiers are related so that the net gain through the limiter remains constant. The distortion products introduced by the nonlinear element are removed by a subsequent filter. The limited, distortion-free outputs of each channel are then mixed, amplified, and then presented to the listener via a transducer. The phase shifts caused by the double bank of filters do contribute distortion to the summed output; however, the processed speech is still highly intelligible.

The most challenging case we have tried to "fit" with

Audibility and Intelligibility of Speech

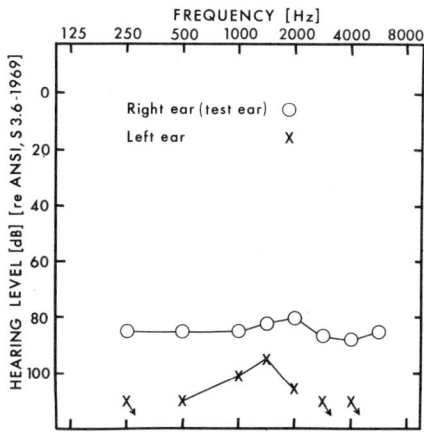

Figure 17. Pure-tone, air-conduction audiogram of the listener with whom we employed the limiting master hearing aid.

the limiting master hearing aid is a listener with a severe, sensorineural hearing loss at the right ear. His audiogram is shown in Figure 17. He has tried 4 or 5 commercial hearing aids, but he has great difficulty understanding words with them. The major difficulty is that it has been impossible to get sufficient gain over a large enough frequency range coupled with the appropriate maximum power output. With the limiting master hearing aid we have been able to achieve this.

Before reporting our results, it is necessary to describe several procedural details. Thresholds of audibility and discomfort were obtained with third-octave bands of noise with center frequencies which coincided with those for the channels of the limiting master hearing aid. To obtain his MCL, the listener is asked to adjust the intensity level of each noise band to the level at which he can obtain the most information and still find comfortable. These threshold and MCL estimates were obtained with a Koss earphone, the same transducer which is employed with the limiting master hearing aid. For the results shown in the next two figures, the output of the Koss earphones was calibrated by placing them on Kemar and measuring the SPL (RMS, slow) with a half-inch condenser microphone and a Zwislocki coupler.[3] The point of reference for the SPL output of the limiting master hearing aid is the microphone placed at the medial end of Kemar's exter-

---

[3] This was the calibration procedure for this set of data. Since there is a significant leak of low-frequency energy and

nal auditory meatus, and not the approximate center of the listener's head in his absence, which was employed in the two studies reported previously.

We have a computer program in which are stored calibrated outputs at each stage within the limiting master hearing aid, including the transducer outputs. In addition, we have stored the word-level contour, which represents the 75th percentile levels of the Pascoe High-Frequency Word List spoken by a male talker at an overall level of 65 dB SPL at the input microphone. With our computer program we can also store a listener's data from noise-band audiometry, and then "add" sufficient gain in each channel to cause the speech inputs to be "amplified" whenever we wish within the listener's dynamic range. We can also set the limiters at or near the threshold of discomfort in each band. From this program we obtain the actual settings for the aid.

The computer printout for this listener's audiometric data, the maximum output intensity levels and the word-level contour for the Pascoe list are shown in Figure 18. The thresholds of audibility are represented by octagons, the thresholds of discomfort by the pluses, the MCL contour by the squares, and the noise floor of the aid by the X's. The word-level contour is parallel to the audibility contour at a 5-dB higher intensity level. The maximum power output is set at the level of this listener's MCL contour. Channels 1 and 2 are turned off. With the aid set in this manner, this listener could not understand any of the ten spondees spoken live-voice by a female talker at 63 dBC (slow meter setting) because they were too soft. Then , the overall gain was raised 13 dB, which caused the word-level contour to be at the threshold of discomfort (see Figure 19). With these settings this listener identified correctly eight out of ten spondees, the highest score he obtained with any which we tried, but he complained that the sound was so loud it hurt his ear. When the overall gain was set 2 dB lower, but the limiter output level was raised 2 dB, the sound was so loud he could not tolerate it. With the overall gain at this same setting, and the limiter-output level at the threshold of discomfort, he identified seven out of the ten words correctly and said that the sound was comfortable. When his own hearing aid was set at MCL, he could only identify 2 out of 10 spondees.

([3] con't.) low reliability for repeated calibration measurements, we are now using a 6-cc coupler attached to a flat plate to calibrate the signal from these circumaural earphones.

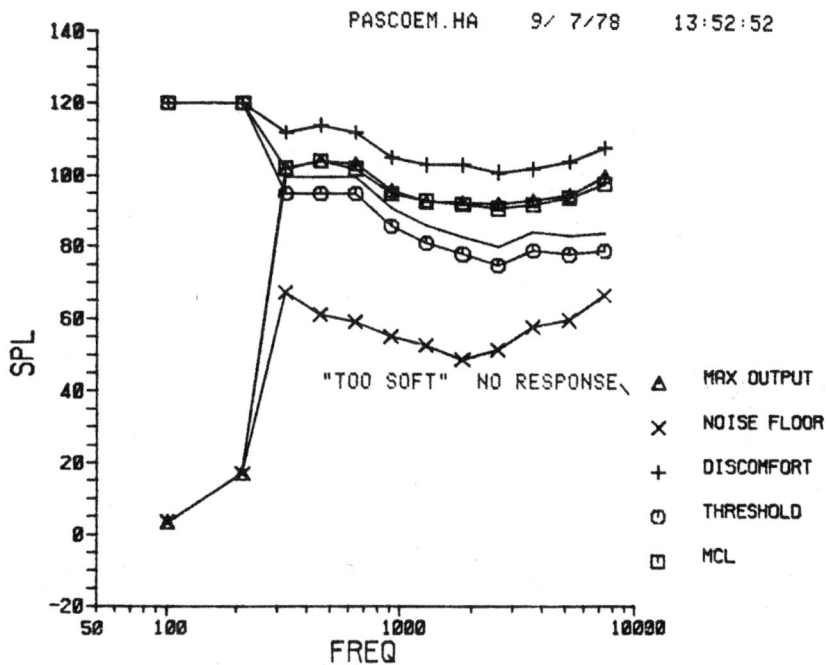

Figure 18. Comparison of the listener's thresholds of audibility and discomfort, as well as MCL with the maximum power output and noise floor of the limiting master hearing aid set 1) to amplify the 75th percentile levels of the Pascoe High-Frequency Word List so that they were 5 dB higher than the listener's threshold and parallel to it, and 2) limit the output at his MCL. When the aid was set in this manner, spondees spoken live voice at 63 dBC (slow meter setting) were too soft for correct identification. The point of reference for the measurement of SPL was the medial end of Kemar's external auditory meatus. Third-octave-band analysis was employed.

It is clear that the parameters of amplification must be exquisitely chosen for him to understand speech best. His best performance is limited by his minimal capability for processing auditory signals. However, the auditory cues, provided with the limiting master hearing aid in subsequent sessions of auditory training, enabled him to communicate with much more ease that with his own hearing aid or without an aid.

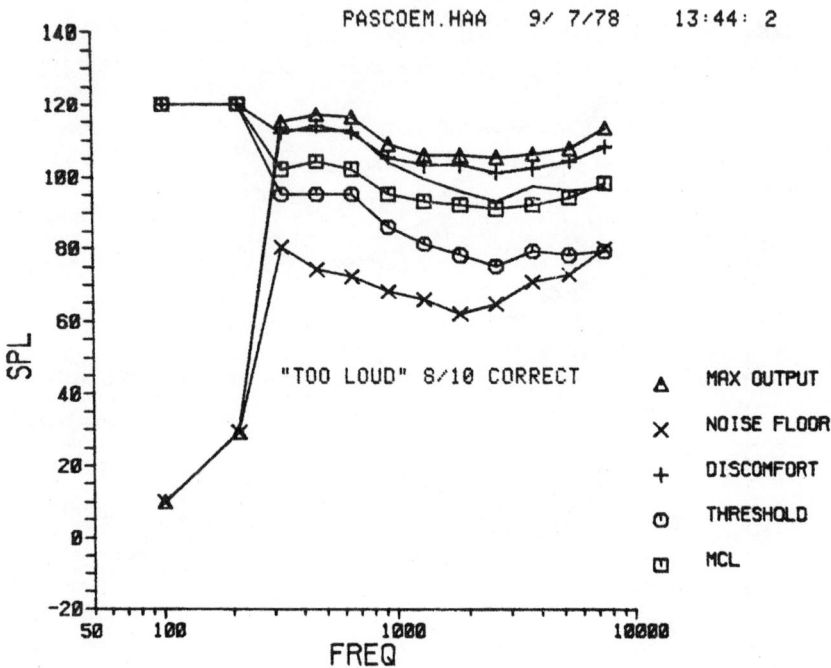

Figure 19. Comparison of the listener's thresholds of audibility and discomfort, as well as MCL with the maximum power output and noise floor of the limiting master hearing aid set 1) to amplify the 75th percentile levels of the Pascoe High-Frequency Word List so that they were 13 dB higher than in Figure 18, and 2) limit the maximum power output at 3 dB above his threshold of discomfort. When the aid was set in this manner, this listener identified 8 out of 10 spondees correctly, but he complained that the sound was so loud, it hurt his ear. The point of reference for the measurement of SPL was the medial end of Kemar's external auditory meatus. Third-octave-band analysis was employed.

Summary

We view the results reported here as exploratory, not definitive. We have tested a limited number of hearing-impaired listeners, and used a single word list in quiet with an arbitrary procedure for analyzing these speech stimuli. Nevertheless, this method of comparing a physical description of the spectral distribution of speech energy with each listener's dynamic range appears fruitful for understanding the relation between 1) the frequency-response, gain and output-limiting characteristics of amplification, and 2) the speech intelligibility of the hearing-impaired listener. This understanding serves as a basis for choosing successive sets of parameters to evaluate in our search for the optimum characteristics.

Several trends do seem significant. Frequency-selective amplification and output-limiting are essential for maximum intelligibility and comfort. It appears that for listeners with sensorineural hearing loss, there is a small range of overall intensity levels which are optimum, and this range becomes smaller the greater the hearing loss and the narrower the dynamic range.

Before we can develop a clinical procedure which is applicable to patients with all kinds of hearing losses, it is essential to obtain much more data from listeners with 1) different types of losses (that is, mixed, sensory and neural), 2) different degrees of losses, and 3) different audiometric configurations, employing a variety of listening conditions (that is, various speech materials and competing signals). The effect of auditory learning through daily experience with a wearable master hearing aid also should be explored. At the same time we need to determine the best signals and psychophysical method to employ for obtaining the thresholds of audibility and discomfort amd MCL. Then these data need to be related to the speech intelligibility scores associated with various frequency-response, gain, and output-limiting characteristics to determine what configuration(s) optimize speech intelligibility for the individual listener. Furthermore, the average speech input levels which most closely approximate those monitored at the microphone of the hearing aid need to be measured. Clinical necessity dictates that procedures for hearing aid fitting and evaluation be based on integration of the best information possible. At the same time, a parallel effort must be made in basic research to improve 1) our strategies for optimizing the frequency-response, gain, and output-limiting characteristics of hearing aids, and 2) the design of hearing aids for hearing-impaired listeners.

Acknowledgment

The preparation of this manuscript and the research described was supported by Program Project Grant No. NS 03856 from the National Institute of Neurological and Communicative Disorders and Stroke of the U.S. Public Health Service.

References

Barth, M.W., Heidbreder, A.F., Niemoeller, A.F., Miller, J.D. and Skinner, M.W., Master hearing aid II., Periodic Progress Report No. 20, Central Institute for the Deaf, St. Louis, Mo., 44, (1978).

Barfod, J., <u>Multichannel compression hearing aids: Effects of recruitment on speech intelligibility</u>. The Acoustics Laboratory, Technical University of Denmark, Report No. 11., (1976).

Barfod, J., Christensen, A.Th., and Pedersen, O.J., Design of hearing aid frequency response for maximum speech intelligibility of patients with high-tone loss. Scand. Audiol. Suppl. 1. 55-60 (1971).

Committe on Electro-acoustics, <u>Hearing aids and audiometers</u>. London: Medical Research Council, Special Report Series No. 261, HMS Office. (1947).

Fowler, E.P., The recruitment of loudness phenomenon. Laryngoscope, 60, 680-695 (1950).

Jerger, J.F., Shedd, J. and Harford, E.R., On the detection of extremely small changes in sound intensity., A.M.A. Arch. Otolaryng., (Chicago) 69, 200-211 (1959).

Lippmann, R.P., The effect of amplitude compression on the intelligibility of speech for persons with sensorineural hearing loss. Ph.D. thesis (Mass. Institute of Tech.) (unpublished). (1978).

Mantovani, M., Pascoe, D.P. and Skinner, M.W., Thresholds of audibility and discomfort, and most-comfortable loudness level of third-octave bands of noise presented in the field. Periodic Progress Report No. 21, Central Institute for the Deaf, St. Louis, Mo., 42-43 (1978).

Mantovani, M., Skinner, M.W., and Pascoe, D.P., Further explorations of the effects of frequency response and overall gain on speech identification in sensorineural hearing loss., Periodic Progress Report No. 21, Central Institute for the Deaf, St. Louis, Mo., 43 (1978).

Pascoe, D.P., Frequency responses of hearing aids and their effects on the speech perception of hearing-impaired subjects. Ann. Otol. Rhin. Laryng. Suppl. 23, 84, 1-40 (1975).

Pascoe, D.P., An approach to hearing aid selection., Hearing Instruments 29 12-16, and 36 (1978).

Skinner, M.W., Speech intelligibility in noise-induced hearing loss: Effects of high-frequency compensation. Ph.D. thesis (Washington University) (1976).

Skinner, M.W., Speech intelligibility in noise-induced hearing loss: Effects of high-frequency compensation. submitted to the J. Acost. Soc. Amer., (1979).

Chapter 11

Summary of the Proceedings of The Symposium on the Application of Signal Processing Concepts to Hearing Aids

Joseph P. Millin, Ph.D.

I assume the audience knows I am supposed to gather general impressions from the proceedings of this conference and to comment on them. I came, therefore, with only a preparatory set, pen and paper. There were difficulties in doing this. One was that the program is so tightly packed that there has been little time to reflect on everything that has been said here. Another is that the range of topics has been so great that it has not been easy to relate the presentations to each other in any cohesive fashion. Nonetheless, I have some impressions that suggest certain directions in which audiology is moving.

Dr. McCandless remarked to me that some of the concepts undergoing current examination are, in fact, rediscoveries or reapplications of earlier discoveries. One of these is the renewed interest in the range of hearing aid response as opposed to thirty years of preoccupation with mid range frequency response. This is evidenced on the one hand by the deliberate suppression of low frequencies as discussed by Yanick and Skinner. While Wegel and Lane dealt only with the effect of tones on tones, it is now generally assumed that excessive amplification of low frequencies will generate a so-called "upward spread of masking" which can obscure or obliterate information, particularly in the critical 1200 to 2500 Hz high frequency region, thus providing drastic reduction in speech intelligibility.

At the opposite end of the speech spectrum, there is a growing conviction that many impaired ears can derive important benefit from added high frequency response, especially in the range from 2500 to perhaps 8000 Hz, which in the past has been regarded as outside the critical range for speech intelligibility.

On the other hand, Yanick raises the issue of whether, in some patients high frequency enhancement might not produce some kind of interference or competition between segments of the auditory mechanism with relatively intact analytic capability and segments with severely reduced analytic capacity. The implication is that in some persons the more severely defective regions of the cochlea have somehow lost their ability to deliver decodable signals to the auditory cortex, while in other patients with similar pure tone losses, the system has somehow retained this coding ability. The latter presumably would benefit from high frequency enhancement of the speech signal while the former would not. This idea is not new, and I seem vaguely to recall speculations by Hirsh about whether the analytic integrity of the high frequency system might differ substantially among patients with comparable, severe high frequenct hearing losses.

While I cannot say whether such dramatic differences do occur, I do think it has become a testable hypothesis and can readily think of several experimental procedures by which it might be tested. Clearly it is a question whose resolution would have dramatic clinical implications for hearing aid fitting.

I find it extremely interesting that Dr. Siegenthaler found evidence of a possible similar binaural phenomenon. That is, in binaural listening, if a poorly performing ear is occluded so that the speech signal reaches only the better ear, discrimination improves. We have two propositions then, a possible monaural interference between functional components of a single ear and a binaural interference between ears. If we add to this some of Jerger's findings of effects produced by improper ear selection or aid placement relative to external competing message or noise sources, a whole new set of promising fitting principals based on these interactions appears to be possible.

It would also appear that on line (real time) pre-processing devices as hypothesized by McCandless and Drucker would offer a major means of minimizing the effects of contaminating sources which degrade signal intelligibility. I mentioned last year the dramatic improvement in speech discrimination scores I obtained by permitting listeners to attenuate, with a multifilter (spectrum shaper), bands within the speech spectrum that were overloaded by certain semi steady noises like typewriter noise or electric drills.

This brings me to another issue, an assumption which has

been stated in audiologic writings, but with which I do not
agree, and that is the the major goal of signal processing is
to reshape the speech signal in a manner which makes the processed signal resemble as closely as possible what normal
listeners would hear without processing. The simple fact is
that there are countless circumstances in which normal ears
hear very badly. This amplifier into which I am speaking at
this moment clearly serves to process the signal for better
understanding than can be achieved by the unaided normal ear.
Despite its non-portability and field coupling, it is in every
sense a hearing aid. Needless to say, perhaps, an environment
which degrades speech intelligibility for normal listeners
must produce devastating effects on the impaired listeners
hearing success. Speech processors offer possibilities for
improvement in signal quality for both normal and hearing impaired listeners.

The work of both Studebaker and McCandless has succeeded
in dramatically improving both the accuracy and precision of
specifying hearing aid performance. The computer modelling
system Studebaker describes offers precise control and manipulation of amplifier performance in the laboratory, and ultimately in the clinic and workaday world. This control has
major importance in our effort to relate instrument performance to listener performance. It is the establishment of
this relation that is the central problem in hearing aid
evaluation, and we have been severely criticized for our failure to do this convincingly. Unfortunately, critics seem
often not to appreciate the complexities of the problem.

Dr. Studebaker summed it up very well in that one little
block on his diagram labelled GOAL. Given that we can have
hardware with any electroacoustic capability we want, how do
we decide what we want? To answer this question we need several things. First we must be able to precisely specify the
auditory parameters of a patient's hearing. We have, fortunately, many measures of these parameters, although I anticipate that others will need development for this specific purpose. Our second requirement is precise control and specification of instrument performance on the patient. This is now
possible as demonstrated by McCandless, Pascoe and Studebaker.

The third step, of course, is to manipulate instruments
and listeners, seeking predictable relations between the two.
The problem to date, as yet largely unresolved, is to find
measures which will clearly reflect the effect of hearing aid
differences on listeners. The need for such measures is
clearly implied in Studebaker's description of a manipulable
or programmable master hearing aid. Having achieved precise
control and measurement of hearing aid performance, compara-

tive procedures can then be used to identify optimum electroacoustic parameters.

It is clear the Dr. Pratt is impressed by the new emphasis on precise measurement and specification of hearing aid performance in the ears of clinical patients. However, as Studebaker implied, this is only half the problem. Let me use an analogy. The speedometer in my car is probably accurate within only three or four miles an hour. To offset the drudgery of long freeway driving I, like most of you I suspect, like to play with the relationships between time and distance. Now that I have two relatively accurate measurement capabilities, a crystal control clock and measured mile markers, I can recalibrate my speedometer. One method is to set my car speed constant at 60 miles per hour and measure the time between markers, from which I calculate my actual speed. It proved to be, after painful mental calculation, only 58.6 miles per hour. Trivial as this may seem, the next step is to establish such questions as braking distance at various speeds, accelleration, safe cornering speeds, passing time and safe driving speeds. In other words, a precise knowledge of how fast my car is going is of no value of itself unless I can make some use of this knowledge. Knowing that I am going ninety miles an hour does not tell me whether this is a safe speed. In like manner, knowing precisely what the sound pressures are at a listener's ear does not tell me whether these are the optimum pressures for speech understanding. So precision of measurement and specification of ear levels is of no value unless I can use this information to determine what these pressures ought to be.

Now that we can precisely specify and control both instrument performance and measures of hearing deficit, we can begin to systematically relate the two, seeking stable, specifiable relations which will enable accurate prediction of optimum fitting for listeners with various audiometric threshold contours, various loudness or tolerance abberrations and various listening environment problems.

The critical problem, however, is still that we must somehow translate these non speech measures into predictors of speech listening ability. No matter how precisely I can measure hearing aid performance, I must be able to specify at some point, not only how performance relates to non speech stimuli, but how these non speech relationships relate in turn to socially adequate speech understanding. I note with interest that both Pascoe and Studebaker acknowledge the need to utilize speech measures to confirm this relationship. Jerger also relies on such speech measures. This does not, in my judgement, mean that we will always need to perform comparative speech measures on every clinic patient, but rather that we must, in the laboratory, use speech measures and possibly also subjective judgments of hearing aid users to translate discovered relationships between non speech hearing aid-patient perfromance to daily patient communication. Once this is achieved we can, with confidence, predict speech listening performance from non speech measures. Then and only then will the goal in Dr. Studebaker's block diagram be specifiable.

Another notion emerging from this conference is the possibility that appropriate hearing aid performance be dynamic. I reject the notion that a single frequency response will produce optimum speech intelligibility as a patient moves from one listening environment to another. This is clearly evident when patients report comfortable, easy speech comprehension in a sound room, but complain immediately of noise when they step out of the room into the hall. Twenty years ago most hearing aids had user adjustable low cut switches, and many listeners used them regularly. Harford, for example, reported that this low frequency attenuation was preferred by many listeners in certain noisy environments, but when the listener returned to a quiet environment, he found the lack of low frequency response to be unpleasant and preferred restoration of low frequency response.

In modern audio reproducing systems, so called equalization networks are commonplace. Something like this, where listeners could readjust the response from one environment to the next seems to me to be desirable if as yet impractical. However it is ultimately achieved, I am convinced that most listeners will be found to require several response options as they move from one place to another. I doubt that current compression systems can provide ongoing response alterations of a magnitude needed to compensate for dramatically different listening environments, so manual alteration by the listener will be necessary. For high speech input levels I anticipate a need for low gain, but relatively flat response. For low level input I suspect most listeners will want high frequency emphasis, possibly extended high frequency range with a reasonably flat low frequency response in quiet, but dramatic low frequency attenuation when competing speech or noise is present. Eventually the ability to selectively attenuate segments of the spectrum seems to me to offer genuine promise. These conclusions seem easily defensible in light of what has been said out at this conference.

With respect to Dr. Vargo's remarks on counseling, some vivid memories were evoked by his presentation. Several psychologists have concluded that the hearing impaired do not differ significantly from the normal hearing population in psychic status, and that the incidence of psychosis or neurosis is about the same in these populations. It has always been my conviction, however, that this conclusion suffers from erroneous sampling techniques. Subjects for such studies have often come from clinic populations, that is, people who were receiving service from speech and hearing specialists. I contend that such persons have already worked through their psychic disturbances, and that resolution of these problems is often necessary before the hearing impaired will even seek assistance. My evidence for this comes from my experience as a hearing aid dispenser. Unlike many traditional audiologists my patients had a continuing relation with me and I got to know them very well. Commonly they would talk about their agony and despair when they first learned of their hearing problem. Many expressed contemplation of suicide and many actually attempted it. Had they been tested at that critical point in time, before they sought help, I suspect that significant psychic disturbance would have been found. In any event, as Steve points out, there are prevalent attitudes among the hearing impaired which require modification if successful use of amplification is to occur.

Finally, many speakers emphasized that electronic engineers have developed capabilities far beyond our knowledge of what to do with them. I have repeatedly insisted that if engineers could give us anything we want we would be hard put to tell him what we want for a particular patient. We are rapidly approaching the time when we can have any reasonable speech processing capability in a wearable device, yet even the simplest questions about appropriate frequency response, band width, compressor functions, the value of frequency transposition, output limitation and other fitting options remain unanswered. In my judgment, this conference has served to identify fruitful avenues for further investigation.

Chapter 12

Panel Discussion
Hearing Aid Selection, Fitting, and Post-Fitting Procedures

Moderator
Joseph P. Millin, Ph.D.

Audience member: It is very important to be able to compress the exact output at specific frequencies in order to help a patient hear better, but is there any option available to me to be able to compress at certain frequencies on a hearing aid?

Dr. Skinner: When we first started looking into the overload phenomenon we were very much concerned that there would be sufficient differences between frequencies that frequency selective limiting might be essential. I still think to a degree that may be true because if you do equal loudness contours up to and including the loudness discomfort threshold level you don't get a straight line in Sound Pressure. It is slightly tilted. But from a practical point of view I'm less anxious about that than I was. I honestly believe you can use almost a straight S.S.P.L. and not sacrifice much dynamic range. It is not as dramatic, let us say, as altering the frequency response. If, however, you have a narrow dynamic range, as you saw with the studies this morning, then I think subtle modification of this, down the road, may be very helpful to squeeze out 2-7 or 8 dB increases in the usable dynamic range at specific frequencies.

Audience member: I fit hearing aids too and I'm concerned with what I can actually take back to make my daily work load more effective. I am aware of a couple of manufacturers that are building instruments that can get two frequency modifications, from 1 KHz up and from 1 KHz down - that doesn't look quite like the arrangement that Dr. Skinner was talking about this morning - but I feel a little frustration as I now realize what it looks like in the research situation as opposed to what it looks like when I look through the manufacturer's specification books. I don't believe there is anything available on the market but I'd love to know if there might be and I'm also interested in an aid that we might be able to use with more variables than just frequency response.

Mr. Yanick: There are no multi-channel hearing aids on the market but there are some hearing aids that permit you to adjust the overall frequency response and compression function. One in particular that is very versatile and flexible is the Widex hearing aid. There is a control panel that permits adjustment of frequency response, output levels and compression function. This can be further modified by acoustic means. In other words, changing vents, using damping elements, various filters and of course earmold modifications.

Audience member: Does it have one frequency control panel, or is it broken down into octaves? I mean, we all have various couplers to use and we can also modify the depth of penetration into the canal or the vent; I'm looking for electronic modifications.

Dr. Millin: Well, one thing that we are all overlooking is that if you have some notion as to what modifications you want initially you can literally order by design what you want as a starting point and achieve modification after that, sometimes by acoustic means. We have a number of instruments in our clinic that have frequency selectivity. I think there may be more of them than you think, possibly.

Audience member: We were talking about single potentiometers. For example, Dr. Skinner was talking about breaking down into 8 or 9 bands of amplification.

Dr. Millin: Oh, I see. That's quite a ways off yet.

Audience member: I'm interested in views on what techniques should be used in clinical fitting. Some time ago in my clinic we started measuring gain in the ear just by simply using the impedance meter or free field thresholds and so on. It seems to me that if you do that you bypass the need for master hearing aids and all this sort of thing. Yet some people seem to be interested in using master hearing aids in the clinic situation. It seems to me you can just bypass all of that and do the sort of thing that is very similar to what Dr.

Hearing Aid Selection, Fitting, and Post-Fitting Procedures

McCandless is doing. I wonder if someone has a view on whether we are missing out on something by not using master hearing aids or anything like that?

Dr. Studebaker: I would start off by passing the buck a little bit. I recently made a review of methods and I don't have a method of my own so I don't think I have any particular biases in this regard but I attempted to analyze what I thought were the elements of a complete method of selecting a hearing aid considering all the various factors that were involved and it was my conclusions that the method that David Pascoe presented last year in Hearing Instruments is that method, at least at this point in time. There's no doubt that in matters of detail that he himself knows that there could be improvements but I still think that that method comes closest to meeting needs clinically and I think that David should comment.

Dr. Pascoe: In considering what can be done with the available hardware, I think it is indispensible that we measure the output of the hearing aid on the person's ear. Also plot the individual's dynamic range both in threshold of discomfort and comfort. You could follow Dr. Berger's analysis of the Australian type of threshold type formulas which assume some suprathreshold relationships. We are now testing both the thresholds, the comfort and discomfort in the same event at the same moment. We are trying to plot that and then we are testing with hearing aids, especially when people come in dissatisfied with their hearing aids. We have a lot of clientele of that sort. People come in to us and say "I have been using this hearing aid for 2 or 3 years and I'm not very happy with it and I've heard you people do some terribly good things" or something like that and "can you tell me if there's a better hearing aid?" And we usually, after doing what I just said, plotting this person's dynamic range which is usually the first time its been done to this person and measuring the output of his hearing aid both on the coupler and on his ear in terms of aided and unaided thresholds and comfort and discomfort aided and unaided and as we send him away for a break so that we can figure out what we've just done in that hour we can plot and usually see the elements that may be causing disconfort. For instance, high levels of gain at 1000 Hz, that tend to bring both ends of the spectrum to insufficient levels as the man sets his aid at comfort or MPO's that are a little too high (20dB, 12dB or 10dB, not 5 or 6) over what we estimate this person's discomfort levels to be assuming that he's not being over conservative, which he may.

But the fact that he's telling us that when we shout it hurts is a clear indication of the fact that there's some consistency in his statements. I am satisfied that after we do the measurements we pull out information and that if we can, supposing this person's aid has a variable MPO and this has happened repeatedly, we reduce it to a lower level and test for discomfort. We find that we now cannot reach discomfort, that the person will tell us it sounds terrible, this band is obviously distorted. He says it rattles but it's not too loud and if at that level of lowering the MPO he's able to function for normal or slightly above normal speech inputs we may be sort of biasing his opinion but he says "Oh, this is much better, it seems a lot more comfortable". If he has a tone control we may be able to shift some of the emphasis from one area to another. If his earmold is vented or not, we may be able to change that and see what happens but actually see it on the patient if the vent had the effect we were looking for or not. For instance, with the all-in-the-ear aid fittings it has happened several times that by plugging the vent with a piece of putty there are surprising effects on the change of frequency response and the sensation or report that the person gives us in terms of the normality of the sound that he is now receiving.

Audience member: More normal?

Dr. Pascoe: More normal, yes.

Moderator: I just saw that recently where I plugged the vent and there was a complete change in the listeners reaction.

Dr. Pascoe: And when we measure to see what happened the usual effect is a shift in the peak from the area around 1000 Hz to a lower frequency range, say 6-700Hz and this appears to give more richness in the voice of the individual without having taken off the high frequencies. There still is cutoff below that point but we have shifted that response peak. Now we are not necessarily satisfied with the immediate report. For instance, a lady said to me very recently after she was seen by an Audiovox distributor that we were not able to get reduction on the same aid and we were trying to get the dealer to supply a different aid. He placed a cotton block in the hook or horn and he said it had reduced the MPO and the lady said it was very comfortable. The reduction was nil in measurements made. It was maybe a matter of 1-3 dB in MPO but the lady said it was very comfortable. We don't necessarily trust the statements that are immediate. We would like to follow a person and see whether or not it is really a difference or not. In general you can get away from doing something blindly and saying this will help you and not knowing what we did when if we know what we have done we can at least accumulate knowledge and compare it to the results. If we see that we have done something specific to the field of sound that the person is receiving, I feel that we're on the way toward being able to accumulate experiences and knowledge as to the relationship of what we did to the actual functional results.

So it seems that we would like to preach the measurement of the dynamic range of the individual with more than speech, with something that is frequency selective. We have found individuals with extremely narrow dynamic ranges and extremely narrow frequency ranges as though there's a sore frequency spot and it would appear that a person like that should not have sounded in that range, whether its the person in the higher frequencies or the middle frequencies like the person in the slides that had a very narrow frequency range. So I would say that with what we have on hand if we can measure the hearing aid on the person and compare it to his or her dynamic range we should be able to see if we could do something to supply better results. Then, of course, it depends on what your assumptions as to what it is you want to supply to the ear, what kind of input levels are you going to test this with, are you going to use some sort of standard that you say this should be placed here, this is the whole thing about what is the objective or the purpose of our selection process. I'm convinced that we can know more about what we are doing and do even more with what we have on the market.

Moderator: Dave, can I suggest a hypothesis that emerges from what you're saying and have the group reflect on tis? If there's one clear cut thing that we know from articulation functions it is that the higher the sound level up to a point the better the speech discrimination, up to a point of course. Now it would seem to me, and you were talking about this high peak center at 1000 Hz and not enough energy in the side bands which represent really the vowel and consonant kind of separation, would it be a reasonable thing to say that probably at modest input the best frequency response would be that one which would produce the highest sound level for speech and yet still achieve a comfortable listening level? Or put it another way, if you have selected the proper frequency response the patient then has an improvement in dynamic range in the sense that since no particular region in the spectrum is pushing him toward an intolerable level, he's able to boost the gain a trifle and therefore achieve a greater overall speech sound level by virtue of a correct fitting as it were? Does that make sense?

Dr. McCandless: If I understand your statement its..., and I hope I can express this clearly because I'm drawing back for some data that we've gathered several years ago and that is the question of the upper limit of the dynamic range. What would happen if you had a point in the dynamic range to which the person was particularly sensitive? You could reverse that by saying what if you have a hearing aid which had a peak that would allow a certain amount of energy to go through and again I'm trying to recall some of the data that we've collected earlier - we had hypothesized in a study that that would occur - actually that discomfort would occur if you had one point that exceeded a certain critical loudness. I don't believe that anymore. I believe it's more related not to the fact that one little point may exceed for a temporary or short period of time but rather it's more an integrated function having to do with bandwidth. Dr. Skinner and some of the other studies suggested that it may not be the absolute level, that it's really more bandwidth related than just point related. Now that wasn't too clear.

Moderator: No, I understand you. But now David is saying some people show a very restricted bandwidth, where others do not.

Dr. Pascoe: This lady that Margo showed in her slides actually has discomfort at threshold.

Moderator: Where?

Dr. Pascoe: At 1200 Hz.

Dr. McCandless: Wasn't this the lady that shifted up after instructions?

Dr. Pascoe: No. At this one frequency, as soon as she hears it, she says that's uncomfortable. Below that she doesn't respond.

Dr. Skinner: That's right. That's the one we shifted with the central notch.

Moderator: I wasn't thinking so much of a sharp resonant peak but simply of a molding of the total response in such a way that it essentially devised the dynamic range and by doing

Hearing Aid Selection, Fitting, and Post-Fitting Procedures 197

that, it would seem to me, provide an elevation of sound level at comfortable listening levels.

Dr. Skinner: Clarify what you mean by increasing the sound level?

Dr. Millin (moderator): What I mean is, let's take a badly misfit hearing aid in which we have an excess of low frequency response and a slope downward. Some of the speech stimuli which are very strong lows and/or noise stimuli in the environment presumably are going to trigger a discomfort level fairly quickly and at fairly low levels. The patient, therefore, in order to get over this intolerable situation will obviously turn down the gain. Now if I contour that so that I divide the range in such a way that that effect does not occur at low levels he can now boost it up another 5 dB, let's say, and he has as much comfort as he had before but we know one thing....Increase sound level, that is to say, raise the total energy of speech above the threshold assuming that there's no severe problem like the woman that you mentioned Dave, and discrimination or intelligibility should improve and I'm saying that the total energy under that curve can be distributed in such a way that all of the speech elements can be elevated above the threshold and a certain minimum amount of elevation necessary to discriminate speech sounds.

Dr. Skinner: Right. I think that it's possible that for a sensorineural hearing loss that you want to get the speech stimulus up to the upper parts of the MCL range for maximum intelligibility at those frequencies.

Dr. Millin (moderator): But it's still got to be comfortable for them.

Dr. Skinner: But it's still got to be comfortable. And I think I agree with Dr. McCandless that it's a total sound stimulus rather than a single band.

Dr. Millin (moderator): Right, but I really had that in mind. That maybe the ideal frequency response shaping would be one that would allow us to get everything that's necessary for intelligibility above threshold sufficiently with the reservation unlike this thing.... I don't know how many of you are aware of the fact that aids tend to be peaked at 1000 Hz and they do have the effect of jamming all the energy right in the transitional range and depressing both the vowel and the consonant content. I think there's something to that. I think maybe a slight dip in the middle might by helpful in separating those ranges and avoiding masking effects and interference.

Audience member: Dr. McCandless talked a minute ago about by setting the maximum output in dB by using the acoustic reflex. Are you using that sort of procedure yourself and is it a fairly hectic procedure? I have two cases myself where I can't get a response and it seems like it might be appropriate.

Dr. McCandless: This could trigger an involved answer which I'll try to avoid. You have to make certain assumptions that we haven't really dealt with and perhaps don't want to here about the dynamic range. One of the assumptions is that we don't have to make assumptions about the thresholds because it's defined but we do have to make assumptions about the upper lid which we have not defined and which, as far as I'm concerned, are as critical, maybe even more critical, as the other ones. With that said, you need to ask the next question. How well does the acoustic reflex represent that upper range or how does it relate to your upper range? In other words, it doesn't have to be precisely that but does it in any way relate to this upper range of usable hearing? That's really the question at hand. In my opinion, there is, as I indicated yesterday, only one reason for limiting, to avoid discomfort. I want to emphasize that. I think we slid over it and it may be the least important reason of all the reasons to limit, but one reason to limit is discomfort. Another reason is to avoid overload or distortion which we don't know how to measure yet but which I think was shown beautifully for the first time in Dr. Skinner's slides, where as you approach the discomfort threshold, discrimination drops down. As you get louder discrimination drops which means to me as you overload the system, distortion products go up. And we know that cochlear distortion occurs. The third reason to limit is to avoid damage. We know that temporary threshold shifts beginning at almost exactly the same levels at least within 5-6 dB. So we're really talking about this same general level in the general range of the acoustic reflex, so it depends on what you use for the stimulus for the reflex whether you assume that that represents the beginning or some sort of upper limit in general. In answer to your question, I believe that it is. I believe that it's a threshold of distortion or breakdown. It's a very natural phenomenon and it's not atypical. Occasional reflexes don't hurt anybody and should be allowed through hearing aids, but any tonics or sustained sorts of things do represent chronic overloads and if you measure it this way, of course, from very nice to some point of subjective, if not loudness, irritability, penetrating, piercing sensation which may not even be in the loudness realm, so yes, I think it's a valid, very helpful technique with children and adults. One reason is because of this instructional problem. If you look at the variances of all the studies and the variances of the reflex there's no question that the reflex measures are stable. They're constant and related to something and if you believe that then I would say yes, they can be used validly.

Dr. Millin (moderator): I just have to comment on something comical that happened to me. If you are aware of the Berger formula, initially he was dividing the threshold loss by 2 at 4000 Hz and adding and saying that's what the gain should be and I discovered that if a person had a 60 dB loss at 4000 Hz and you gave him 30 dB gain with an input signal on the speech spectrum that was only 30 dB but the output was 60 dB or right at threshold and though you gave him his gain an ordinary speech signal is never audible. So I see some dangers in manipulating numbers like that without finally making the pressure measurements in the ear to a real stimulus to find out what you got. You can have gain at 4000 Hz but theoretically at ordinary conversation level nothing over threshold ever comes in at that frequency. So he dropped a number, pretty small, 1.3 or2 or something like that in order to get some energy in that was actually audible according to his own theory that he was fitting to a speech spectrum rather than a flat response. These are the kinds of things that Dave said, whenever you get a patient in and you look at what they've got you suddenly discover, yes, they have gain at 4000 Hz but they're not hearing anything there. And I just wanted to throw that in.

Audience member: It occurs to me that the vast majority of hearing aid fittings that I've done, I took one of the standard or classic hearing aid fitting techniques and I find very many people are satisfied but there are those people who have problems. I think we touched on this earlier. I'm wondering whether you people are suggesting that we should incorporate all these kinds of technologies into our standard hearing aid evaluations or that we can continue to do regular hearing aid evaluations reasonably successfully?

Dr. Vargo: I'm glad you asked that. Because it was precisely what Joe and I were discussing earlier or as a matter of fact between the break this afternoon. I think there's a danger in the assumption that "satisfaction" can be equated with optimal performance in terms of our criterion measure which happens to be word discrimination. We should not simply equate them on a one to one relationship. I am amazed personally and I'm sure many of the panel are that as many people as have been "misfitted" still can be classified as satisfied users of hearing aids when in fact their optimal performance may never have really been approached.

Dr. Studebaker: I'd comment on that same question that there's a distinct difference between much of the research that you've heard the last few days and that which has been published on what's the optimum response a hearing aid ought to have. There's a difference between that kind of research and how one might go about various aspects of fitting a hearing aid and an actual clinical method that's complete. I don't think it's the responsibility of people in the field actually working with patients to take the raw research output of various projects, as good as they might be, and attempt to work those into a clinical procedure of their own and that's why I think that some of the published methods need to be evaluated for their completeness as clinical methods. I think a good example of the differences between these two kinds of studies or published reports is characterized by the two papers that David Pascoe wrote. His own dissertation is an example of research results that tells you something about the relationship between frequency response and hearing loss. Dr. Skinner's is another one. David's report last summer in Hearing Instruments on how to go about getting a real hearing aid on a real person is the second kind and I think that second kind is the type you need to be paying attention to now and people making up those methods need to think about the basic research results that come from the other studies.

Audience member: It is my understanding that Dr. Pascoe used narrow bands of noise for measurements. Can you use pure tones and get the same information?

Dr. Pascoe: You mean if you use pure tones to do field testing to compare aided vs. unaided?

Audience member: Yes.

Dr. Pascoe: Well, it may be more preferable to use something other than just straight pure tones, maybe a warble tone may be more effective depending on the type of room that you're using to test in. Whether you have a room that is relatively small and hard-walled. For instance, most of the pre-built booths are not necessarily very good for field testing. Whether you're using a larger room where the elements of the room block whats on the screen, whether that room can be a little ignored or not makes the difference on whether you can use pure tones or not. If you can use a signal that you can be certain is not variable with minor movements of the head of the listener, which is the problem with pure tones, whether he's really listening to the signal or he's turning up and down. If you have a steady signal then you can use it. You have to have a sound level meter to follow the level of the signal on the listener's ear or its proximity to see if you can use it wherever you are. I have never been able to successfully test with straight pure tones. I have been forced to try them in different countries where I have had seminars and it's very difficult to obtain repeatable results on free field tests with pure tones as far as I'm concerned. I have had measurements of hearing aids in classrooms with pure tones coming from audiometers because there was no other equipment available and I've had a hard time repeating the same frequency response twice in uncontrolled situations. We like the noise band simply because of their greater diffusion and lower response to a small type of head movement.

Dr. Millin (moderator): It has some effect on the aid, too, Dave, because at some frequencies the aid may never have enough very rapid change that you'd see on the slope of some regions whereby a broader range will sample a larger segment of the hearing aids response. We have used a compressor to maintain the level in the room. Now that's a very complex thing and we're just doing that experimentally, but we have actually put a little microphone on the ear and let it monitor and control the level coming in and adjust it on the compressor and use that as an audiometric thing but that's a complex procedure and only really a laboratory thing right now.

Dr. Skinner: Could I make one more comment? I'd like to tell you that at CID although in the clinic we're using an instrument built in our lab to generate the third-octave bands of noise, in the research that I'm doing right now we've recorded the third-octave bands of noise. We're using a high quality tape recorder where we get approximately a 50 dB signal-noise ratio and we've set the filters for recording our bands of noise at a greater than 60dB/octave skirt. So that we're getting good resolution of that third-octave band and it's possible that what we really ought to do at CID is generate some tapes and make them available for use in your clinical situations. Does that sound like a feasible way to go?

Dr. Millin (moderator): The only comment I'd like to make and I was hoping Geary would respond to this is a thing you may have overlooked and I meant to mention it when I spoke earlier and that is that despite the inherent differences in many of these methods if you'll look at the derived results they are incredibly similar at times.

Dr. McCandless: My comment at lunchtime was that I like to see things simplistically because it's the only thing I can handle and just looking over all the things said here and in recent literature, as far as the manufacturers are concerned there seems to be more convergence on the things that are being done derived from a variety of different ways than I've ever seen in my professional career. I don't know how the others feel. By that I mean that the results that you saw here were very much like Berger's ½ rule, very much like the technique that we use, very much like some of the things that were even reported twenty years ago. But they are generally supportive and not contradictory. They fit with Sam Lybarger's computations of a few years ago in general. What I'm saying is I think there's a convergence of measurements despite what stimuli are used, despite understanding the effects of couplers and so forth, to a degree that we've never had before. We're very, very close to this transitional point between making some valid, useful techniques for placing the hearing aid on the subject. I agree it may not be here but it's closer than it has ever been.

Dr. Millin (moderator): I think you get a lot of similarity between the results of the various methods if you compare the results of what we get from each other.

Audience member: I want to ask Dr. Skinner if she ever made a comparison between the free field measurement with the third-octave band to an influence to get a relationship not with a hearing aid but to an ear itself?

Dr. Skinner: I have not done that but David has. You made a conversion, didn't you, with the third-octave band?

Dr. Pascoe: Well, we were comparing thresholds at both receivers with standard ear molds, light ear molds, over the ear with MX-41 type cushions in field and we had some averages for a group of 20 young listeners. The results are very similar to what you would have if you were to compare the ANSI standards as a MAP measurement and a MAF measurement in which the hearing threshold at 3000 Hz is in the neighborhood of -2dBSPL compared to a 10dBSPL on the ANSI which makes it a 12dB difference there and about -3 or -4dB at 4000 Hz which makes another 12-13 dB difference and then the problems of the lower frequency range where the cushion leakage is absent in the field testing so that if the ANSI is 25 dB standard at 250 Hz, and 45dB at 125 Hz in the field it may be something like 38 at 125 and 21-22 at 250, with the middle frequencies being very coincident. Is that what you were asking?

Audience member: I would like to ask you with your procedures if you notice any difference when people report tinnitus? Do you notice any problems either to fit them?

Dr. Pascoe: People, especially when your pure tone testing, will report that "that tone I had difficulty responding to because it always seems to be there and I get mixed up". That's a very common statement from listeners when you're testing between 3000 to 6000 Hz. So we usually proceed to do a pulsed tone comparison so that this is 'OK, just listen to the one that goes beep-beep-beep and not the long one' type thing in order to help the raising of the hand with more precision. As far as the hearing aid, I have not noticed any problem. In general, I'm very curious about the tinnitus sensation and when I ask them to compare loudness between say a 500 Hz or a 1000 Hz tone and their sensation of tinnitus, I find SL's of 10-15 dB at most and I've never seen any of the reported 30 or 40 dB tinnitus SL's and most of those sensations seem to be quite blocked out by any other sound present in the ear, so I haven't had any trouble with people who are wearing a hearing aid and will say the tinnitus is interfering. Maybe I don't come into contact with that population.

Audience member: I'm sorry that Dr. Pratt has left. I wanted to ask him about the Otometry method he has referred to in his talk which has been proposed as a standard technique. I have not seen any standard research on this technique. Do any panel members have any comments regarding Otometry?

Dr. Millin (moderator): I'm sure you'll get plenty of comments. I just want to say briefly with all his emphasis on precision of measurement he has left out certain information regarding the rationale for it. It is not really possible to perform experiments on it.

Dr. Studebaker: I think there's a nugget of a good idea in Otometry, but it's difficult to extract it. The writings in the area are very difficult to follow. But there is a nugget of a good idea that has yet to be tested to see whether or not, in fact, it is a valid one. The idea of using a signal which has some known loudness in the normal ear as a function of frequency or to use a set of frequencies which have some known loudness relationship to each other, whether equal loudness or some other relationship, it really doesn't matter, can be handled in the technical aspects of how it's applied, and then to attempt to find the most comfortable loudness as you use those signals that are comfortably and equally loud in the normal ear and to present those signals to the person wearing a hearing aid and to adjust the hearing aid until those signals are most comfortable and equally loud in the that ear seems to me to be a reasonable hypothesis; a hypothesis that has yet to be tested for validity, though.

Audience member: Would it be reasonable to assume that if you arrive an at equal or most comfortable level using that signal that it would also be that it would result in the most understanding?

Dr. Studebaker: That's part of what has to be tested. I think that that's the thing which we do not know at this time.

Dr. Millin (moderator): In fact, if you were to look at Posner and Ventry and some of the other studies, you would have to say that comfort level, although there's nothing you can do to prevent the listener from listening at comfort level, does not produce the best speech discrimination scores.

Audience member: Next year I'd love to see more attention given to ear molds. It would be well worth the time and of tremendous benefit. Paul Yanick mentioned single side band clipping. Is there such a thing?

Mr. Yanick: There is a group in England that has a wearable hearing aid with single side band and they've done considerable research on it. We have a prototype that we built down at Monmouth College with dual channel compression and a single side band limiting but nothing that can be worn on the head yet.

Audience member: Paul, you mentioned intermodular distortion yesterday. I spent $4000 on this nice phonic ear computer so I could see why my hearing aid didn't sound right to my ear and there was harmonic distortion. Harmonic distortion is within normal limits and the hearing aid still sounds lousy and after I paid my money I got frustrated and started asking people why it still sounded lousy when harmonic distortion was okay. They suggested it might be intermodular distortion. Is there some way of calculating that sort of consideration?

Mr. Yanick: There is no accepted or standard way to measure intermodular distortion. I think Dr. Millin can answer that more completely.

Dr. Millin (moderator): Actually, with something like the Fry box you can't do this because actually to test intermodular distortion you need two input signals both of which are suppressed in order to look at what is left over. While it's true that in a way the devices measure second harmonic distortion and what they've gone to, to considerable extent now, is suppressing the input frequency and looking at everything that's left over and they sometimes call that second harmonic distortion when it's not. It's total distortion with the assumption that most of it is occurring at the harmonics. You can't do that with what you have. I can think of ways where you could look at it, however, and I'd be glad to talk to you about it. You can do it with the B+K hearing aid test box if you can find two inputs, that is with the more complex type of test box, that gives you more latitude because that not being a computerized device it is not programmed for just one function. But I'm not sure I want to look at clinically until I can demonstrate with certainty what it means. For example, we've tested several receivers and found that they follow the waveform beautifully and yet when you chop them off they stop in 6 or 7 msec. We have found others that have run for 300 msec. That's incredible variation which is some source of a problem. We also did a frequency response on a hearing aid recently in which we got this very high deflection of the needle and we got nice frequency response and when a student says, "Well, what is all that in there?", I said, just looking at the meter, "That hearing aid is just noisy as hell". Yet it had a frequency response that was elevated above the noise. We took it out and put it to our ear and there was high noise, but when you did a so-called 'harmonic distortion' on it you didn't see the noise at all because when you filtered it you knocked 9/10 of it out. So it takes a great deal of sophistication to even identify these problems, but there's no question in my mind but that the noise level generated by that hearing aid was excessive for the listener. It was above his threshold. There's no standard test for this at this time. We should look into it.

Audience member: What do you do about it?

Dr. Millin (moderator): I don't know. Get the aid repaired if it has a lot of noise. I'd say this, if you have that kind of equipment I'd be fussy as hell about the kinds of aids I'd accept into my clinic. You might as well get good ones. Whether you can only test harmonic distortion, or even if you reject the fundamental and look at everything else, if the levels are a little high, send it back. Probably anything you read there is going to relate to other factors like the transient response of the receiver and all other kinds of things.

Since intermodulation distortion is a low frequency phenomenon, that is the products basically come up in the low frequencies and the hearing aid receivers transmit low frequencies rather well, whereas when you have a harmonic distor-situation the distortion products are in the high frequency end the receiver does not transmit them very well, if the distortion products come up above the high frequency cut-off of the receiver you simply don't see them there. If the hearing aid sounds bad with an input signal, chances are it is indeed intermodulation distortion.

Audience member: It might be of interest in as much as intermodulation distortion has been done in so many different ways, it really hasn't been defined as to what you're really doing. There is a new graph in an International Standard on a method of making intermodular distortion that might be a little more meaningful and that will become available in a few months.

Dr. Millin (moderator): And again if you adopt this thing then the thing is to relate it to listener effects.

Audience member: It's a very difficult thing on a hearing aid where you have a certain response to get meaningful results.

Dr. McCandless: It's been observed over the years that there is a very poor relationship between harmonic distortion and intermodular distortion and speech discrimination scores at least assuming that the harmonic and intermodular distortions are within reasonable bounds. And I think that we generated some data recently which would indicate that is not a surprising outcome. One of the reasons it is not surprising is because the basic speech signal is a line spectrum signal and if you think about it a moment you recognize that if the various components of a line spectrum vowel generate harmonic distortion or intermodulation distortion all of those distortion products end up at one of the other lines. And therefore, the only influence it has on the basic vowel spectrum is to change the spectrum shape of the vowel if the distortion is strong enough to add to or subtract from, depending upon its phase relationship, the other line spectra elements and you have to have a whole lot of distortion before significant amounts of spectrum shaping changing occurs.

Chapter 13

Panel Discussion
Cochlear Electrostimulation

Moderator
Lindsay L. Pratt, M.D.

Audience member: Has the phenomenon ever been studied in normal ears? You might have what we would call "super-hearing"?

Dr. Martin: As far as I know, no, it has not been studied in normal ears.

Audience member: Why would you use only 30 hours? It seems that if 30 hours is good, then 60 hours might be better.

Dr. Martin: That may be. The original paper by Puharich and Lawrence proposed 20 hours. The work that has been done clearly showed that 30 hours was better than 20. 30 hours is 6 weeks. Its quite conceivable that if you went further, you'd get more. In fact, what we discovered is that the improvement continues after therapy has been discontinued for a period of at least 2 to 3 months. That is to say, 2 months after therapy there is a statistically significant improvement above the immediate post-therapy tests. So its quite possible, we just haven't done it. This is quite expensive work to do in terms of time. Figure that it takes a month to collect subjects and do pre-testing, at least 2 months for therapy itself, another 2 months for post-testing and data analysis and so on. That's a half a year, so it's very expensive work and that's one reason we haven't tried that yet.

Audience member: The signal you are using is placed on the head, not just on the ears. Has there been any investigation of other parameters in addition to hearing changes that might occur?

Dr. Martin: I think in relation to one particular kind of data that we've gotten that that should be followed up. In fact, we've begun to look at things like blood work related to stress reactions. We have an interesting fact that we've discovered which is that people with sensorineural loss in one ear apparently do not show, in general, appreciable improvement. That's consistent with the view that there's some sort of metabolic situation which has caused a loss in both ears which is in some way being reversed by therapy. So you might expect other physiological effects. It may be that this therapy is very general in its effects and that we have only discovered one of the parameters in the hearing aspect. We just don't know.

Mr. Prout: You asked about other effects and as Dr. Martin pointed out it takes a long time just to evaluate the effects on hearing but along the way we pick up subjective reports from subjects which really just about bend your mind. We have one subject who has atrophied 8th nerves, which means he's getting absolutely nothing from his hearing to his brain. He reported that after a few weeks of therapy that he noticed his lawn mower was noisier. We've had other people, mainly older people, who report that they've been remembering things they've forgotten years ago. This is a common individual report, that long term memory has returned. Now anybody who finds money for research, there's exciting possibilities.

Dr. Studebaker: Yesterday you commented on a pure-tone threshold change that has been observed of an order of magnitude of approximately 15 dB. Please describe this experiment in a little greater detail. What were the tone levels, masker levels, etc?

Dr. Bienvenue: The procedure that was used is a tone-on-tone masking procedure. Its based on the technique developed by Zwicker as reported in 1974 which he called "psychoacoustic tuning curves". Basically what you're doing is setting a signal, we used 2 KHz, and then a Bekesy audiometer is used to generate a masker tone. The subject sets the level of the masker tone so its just barely masking the probe tone. Under those conditions what we're seeing is its change in the rejection of masker, the signal-to-noise ratio, that you can tolerate. But there's a change of up to 15 dB depending on the frequency you're looking at, in the set level of the masker tone given the presentation signal level.

Dr. Studebaker: What's the relationship between the frequency of the masker tones and the frequencies of the test tones?

Dr. Martin: The more remote the masker the larger the difference in the level of masker tolerated. As you get close in there seems to be a smaller difference. I believe you're down to only 5 dB or so when you're getting close in the relatively high frequencies. In the lower frequencies you're seeing a larger difference.

Audience member: What are the frequencies and currents that you actually used on this treatment?

Dr. Martin: There are seven different electrode combinations on this instrument. Two operations where the bare electrodes are applied directly on the skin and the others are combinations of bare and insulated electrodes and the frequency is lowest for the bare electrodes by themselves. I think the lowest carrier is about 7 KHz and the highest carriers with the two insulated electrodes is about 30 KHz.

Audience member: Point of clarification on the amplitude of the nature of the modulation.

Dr. Martin: This is amplitude modulated with a sweeping Bekesy audiometer frequency. It sweeps from about 50 Hz to 10,000 Hz very gradually and then it sweeps back slowly in the other direction. The amplitude of that modulation is also changing by a triangular waveform. We have actually a three dimensional stimulation here.
    One other point on the frequencies of this. The carrier is set at a resonant frequency with the person in therapy. The carrier does vary - it gets up to as high as 50 killicycles.

Audience member: You have indicated that it takes some 2 months or so to establish the therapy and create the effect. How long does the effect last?

Dr. Martin: Well apparently whatever benefit is there remains until very shortly before it drops off. That is, the drop off is rather radical. The onset of improvement is very gradual. People will tell you during therapy, "Well I don't notice any change", and even after therapy when you can show on PB tests that there has been a significant improvement, some people will report no noticeable change. However, I think this is because of the gradual onset. Three months later they will come in and say "My hearing has just gone to pot. Last week it happened", and if you test them they are back to pre-therapy levels.

Audience member: How do you stop that?

Dr. Martin: Its possible to continue therapy. Now we haven't worked out the parameters of this yet. Some people just give it continuously forever. We have obviously considered and we've begun to do some of that type of work to try to reduce the amount of therapy as much as possible and still maintain the effect.

Audience member: When you do therapy again on a subject after he's returned to his pre-therapy condition, does it take it longer or shorter to return to the improvement you originally saw with therapy? Also, do you get more or less improvement? Are there any differences in the effects of the improvement in a second approach to the therapy sessions?

Dr. Martin: It's just about the same. It takes the same amount of time and the return is just to about the same levels.

Audience member: You commented yesterday that on some of the research by Dr. Simmons that different parts of the test sessions were accomplished with different word lists and that the differences in word lists might account for the differences or lack of differences in speech discrimination data. And is it also possible that the lists were not equivalent? You commented that you used the same list on the testing of each person. Is it possible there is a learning effect?

Dr. Martin: At least possible. Well there certainly could be a learning effect and that's the reason for a placebo. Absolutely. You expect placebo effects. And the significances that we reported were in differences between placebo groups and experimental groups, so that you're quite right, there is no doubt that in some of these tests there is some sort of learning effect to take that particular kind of test but you control for that by running a placebo group which, although they think they are getting the therapy, does not get the therapy. They, of course, had the same type of pre- and post-test situations as does the experimental group.

Dr. Drucker: What do you mean by the resonant frequency of the person as included in this system?

Dr. Martin: Let me explain about this resonant frequency. The impedance of the electrodes on the head is capacitive. Inside the machine there are three different sets of inductors that are placed in series with the electrodes. Therefore, the circuit is a series resonant circuit, capacitive through the electrodes and inductive in the machine. This is supplied in the therapy device. This is, in terms of ham radio operators, a master oscillator power amplifier circuit, where the oscillator itself is the power amplifier. The frequency is controlled by the capacity of the electrodes and, as was pointed out before, it can vary as the capacity changes. But this variation is small compared to the shift between modes of operation. With regard to the series circuit, since we have only a 24 volt power supply in the device you might think the voltage was not very high although because it's a series circuit and apparently it's a fairly high cue we have measured voltages on the order of 300 volts on the insulated electrodes. Now you don't get that on your head and you would never feel it because it's operated below the sensation of shock. But the voltages are extremely high in some cases.

Dr. Drucker: So this is not the resonant frequency of the individual, it has something to do with the system?

Dr. Martin: No, it's not an individual physiological resonance.

Dr. Drucker: The system again puts some sort of signal on the individual. It would not be unreasonable to anticipate that the effect could be more global than simply limited to the hearing mechanism. Have you observed other changes than the specific audiometric changes you have discussed?

Dr. Martin: We have done a little bit of work with Evoked Response. Just a look at it. It seems that there might have been something there. We have also begun some work relating to the psychological correlates of stress, psychophysiological correlates of stress, but we haven't done that yet. These are the types of things in progress.

Audience member: In investigating the phenomenon that you are studying it would appear that it might be possible to clarify some of the effects going on by doing animal studies. Have you done any animal studies?

Dr. Martin: Yes, that would be very nice. One of the difficulties of course is the placement of the electrodes. That's hard enough with human beings who are intelligent and know you are not going to destroy them. It's very, very stressful for animals, obviously. There is a possibility that we might move from this type of presentation, using electrodes, to some sort of inductance. But we haven't got the equipment for that right now. Obviously animal studies would be very nice. Why don't you do it? I wish you would.

Audience member: Let me play devil's advocate here. I am on the human subject safety committee for my own institution and what you are saying here is that in describing an experiment using this procedure you are applying a signal of considerably high strength, an electrical signal, to the human subject. How would you reply to the degree of safety of the human subject in this context?

Dr. Martin: We were very concerned with the margin of safety. In fact, for a year now we simply sat with our machines in the laboratory and looked at them and worried about that. Finally, the first paper we did was in conjunction with Dr. Brennan, chief neurologist at Hershey Medical Center and we did a number of electroencephalograms before and after. He felt, clinically, that there was no need to worry about it. There was no evidence, given our findings, that there was any kind of problem and he felt, given the other literature, there wasn't any problem.

Dr. Studebaker: There has been a comment regarding the switchbox for use in these experimental procedures. A switchbox which has multiple setting positions and which you used in the double-blind context, where the subject does not know whether or not they are getting therapy and the person administering the therapy does not know if the person is getting therapy. First of all, are you still using that switchbox, and if you are does the examiner have access to a meter of some sort indicating the resistance across the electrodes or something like that?

Dr. Martin: We are no longer doing double-blind experiments at this time, since as far as we are concerned every well run study has shown positive results. However, we do use a single-blind procedure. Now it's quite possible that the technician ..... we can't say that he does not communicate something to the subject in the placebo conditions. So we use a single-blind placebo group at this point, just to get some idea of what the natural placebo effect would be. The apparatus in the experiment is one in which the placebo subject is experiencing everything that the experimental subject is experiencing in terms of the natural sounds produced in the head by the electrical stimulation. There is a small speaker in the headset which generates those same sounds. The dials, meters on the box, etc., which the subject can see if he wants to, are set up to perform in the same way. The only way he would notice a difference is if suddenly the technician were to take the electrodes off the head and if he were an experimental subject the needles would drop back to 0; if he were a placebo subject, they would not. I don't think that's a real problem, quite frankly.

Mr. Prout: I think that what Jerry's getting at is, that of monitoring the conditions under which the subject is being stimulated during the course of his exposure. Is that what you were getting at? How do you know it doesn't drop off in the course of treatment or his exposure?

Dr. Martin: Yes, of course, we have someone monitoring at all times.

Audience member: What does he see and do if something changes?

Dr. Martin: Well, we have a technician who is trained to handle that sort of thing. He's there all the time making sure the contacts are in place, because if the subject sneezes things might move off. That's a very important part of the therapy.

Dr. Studebaker: I had an opportunity to see the experimental setup of Dr. Hughes a while ago and he was running what was supposed to be a double-blind experiment. However, the technician who administered the therapy was also the audiologist and the technician was able to subjectively guess which subjects were placebo and which were not by observing the meter which indicated whether or not a signal was going to the head of a given subject. This would potentially breech the double-blind nature of the study for the side of the audiometric technician administering therapy and doind testing.

Dr. Martin: In our first experiment, the double-blind experiment, the person who was the technician didn't know there was a placebo group. I don't even think that she knew there were such things. She simply was there and told there were different types of conditions, period. The subjects were told that too. I don't think that it ever occurred to her that there were subjects not receiving therapy. She was simply told to switch each subject to his or her own particular number. And that person was not our audiologist. Our audiologist was, in fact, Gordon Bienvenue who didn't know anything about the study at all and simply came in before and after and put those people in a sound room and did speech discrimination tests.

Audience member: Speaking of side effects - was there any tinnitus as a result of this procedure?

Dr. Martin: We did not find any. Other have reported that, but I can't say.

Audience member: I'm interested in the theoretical mechanism involved in this effect. Is it possible that the effect is changing some sort of metabolic state or potential state of the spiral ganglion, the auditory nerve? Is there a change in the cochlear potential at the outer hair cells, or some similar phenomenon? Is there some theory now regarding what seems to be happening?

Dr. Martin: That's an interesting set of questions and I wish I could say something interesting beyond what I said yesterday. The question which is constantly asked, and quite appropriately, is "Well, what's the mechanism?" What we're sure of, at least for our own work, is that we get the results. We have some information now about the levels of current required for it and what tests show it most appropriately and so on. We're just beginning to explore these other questions, doing blood work and so on, which might show some relation between TD therapy and some other parameters that are apparently involved in threshold shift and so on. But that's just very speculative right now. It's possible we may be changing cell memory potentials, which are known in many cases to be the result of stress. We may also be effecting blood flow.

Dr. Millin: A question regarding the accuracy of describing this signal as being in the radio frequency signal.

Dr. Martin: It's perfectly well qualified to be an electromagnetic spectrum. There are modulated signals as low as 2 to 5 Hz and they still are electro-magnetic. So it qualifies.

Dr. Millin: Concerning the nature of the signal being presented to the subject, Dr.Martin points out that this type of signal may be non-medium bound and therefore, we ask how is the signal transmitted, where does it exist, is it limited to the direct electrical contacts in the system, are you actually creating an electro-magnetic field in the environment and how far might this spread?

Is the head acting as a resistor in the one case, the direct case and is it perhaps acting as an antenna in the non-medium bound condition?

Mr. Prout: I don't believe the head is acting as an antenna. The current is strictly conducted through the head; the head is mostly capacitive as far as the electrodes are concerned. We had no experiments that tell us how deep the signal penetrates through the tissues. We were preparing to do an experiment like that but never got the time or money.

Audience member: Could you by use of this therapy procedure counteract the effects of noise exposure? Could you eliminate or reduce the amount of temporary threshold shift in a noise exposed subject by using the therapy either before or in conjunction with a noise exposure?

Dr. Martin: We have evidence one subject (that's me) and it was negative or we would have done some more. We may try it again.

Dr. Siegenthaler: At the recent International Congress of Audiology in Oklahoma there was considerable attention given to another kind of electrostimulation of the cochlea, under the name of cochlear implants. The current is delivered, one way or another, into the cochlea with various degrees of sophistication, as I was hearing. I don't know the field very well. At one extreme they were sticking a wire into the round window and the other extreme was implanting 12 channels filtered throughout the cochlea. Now, as I understood it, they were using speech or signal input, filtering it into as many channels as they were using and then putting each one of those electric signals directly into the cochlea through these electrodes. What is the relation between that kind of cochlear stimulation which is electrical and this kind of? Are they the same or are they different phenomena? Do we know anything about cylinder effects and so forth? Incidently, the purpose was to make you hear, to be a "hearing aid" and I know of no evidence that it was for long range therapeutic effect.

Dr. Martin: That's the difference. The work on cochlear stimulation is to develop a communication device and this is not. This is an attempt to produce long term and stable changes in the cochlea or hearing system.

Dr. Siegenthaler: Isn't this then a kind of hearing aid of sorts?

Dr. Martin: Well, that was the reason it was discovered. That is to say the attempt was to develop a hearing aid of some sort using the Piazzo electric effect produced by the radio waves. And the finding that people were somehow improving in their hearing was accidental.

Audience member: What you are hearing is not a Piazzo electric effect but an electrophonic effect, essentially bone conduction.

Mr. Prout: What you are going to hear is essentially the effect of a condenser phenomenon. You are vibrating the skin of the head, you are vibrating, ultimately, the bone of the skull and you are hearing essentially bone conduction.

Dr. Martin: That's right, that's what you hear, but in terms of what's placed on the head, it's quite different.
 I'd like to say one thing in regard to the sound sensation that you hear with this machine. We can produce reasonably good stereo with this. It has that difference from bone conduction. We maintain good separation.

Dr. Drucker: There is a difference between an acoustic signal and an electro-magnetic signal. We are placing an electro-magnetic signal on the head in this case, so why should this be the same as bone conduction?

Dr. Martin: But there is a Piazzo electro effect. You do get compression of the tissues under those conditions.

Audience member: I disagree with the use of the word "Piazzo electric". I feel this is basically a phenomenon of electrostatic attraction. What has been called the "electrophonic effect".

Dr. Martin: Maybe so.

Dr. Pratt: Well there's nothing like being a clinician and not knowing what's going on. Does anyone else understand all these terms? I'm very confused. As a clinician I'd love to see this work and I appreciate even more that we in the medical arena are so dependent on people with experiences in many different arenas. Your knowledge has contributed so much to the ultimate care of the patient, but I'm lost.

What about the medical-legal aspects of performance of this therapy?

Mr. Yanick: I'm concerned with the medical-legal aspects in the sense that patients with various forms of fluctuant and progressive sensorineural hearing loss should be evaluated more completely to determine possible cause or aggravating factors associated with their hearing loss. Everything that can be done medically should be done before such a procedure is indicated. The Otologist, in particular, must focus more attention on metabolism and biochemical mechanisms so commonly involved in long term progressive and fluctuant forms of sensorineural hearing loss. It is highly possible that TD therapy in conjunction with treating metabolic and biochemical abnormalities, will yield even better results than Dr. Martin described earlier in his study.

Dr. Pratt: We live in constant fear of medical-legal. After your first lawsuit, you're ego damaged. After your second suit, you're mad. And after your third suit, you say "Here we go again". The reason I say this is, I have one right now. I had a tumor out of a big carotid gland, a huge tumor; I have written on the chart in the office 'facial nerve damage explained'. Then in the hospital chart it's written and in my post-op note it's written what our plans were, but in so far as the patient was concerned, he didn't understand this.

My point being, I don't care what you do medically-legal. It doesn't mean a thing concerning consents. What you have to do, and this is why our premiums are so high, I have to prove my innocence in court, and I think we lose our purpose worrying about medical-legal aspects. We're talking about electro-magnetic waves, etc. No one knows about them. Can you imagine someone getting on the stand and being asked about it? You would be made a fool because the jury doesn't understand you either.

So we try to analyze the problem and try to have committees so the whole committee gets sued instead of one person but we should examine the medical-legal problems but not suppress our research because of it.

Audience member: What about funding?

Mr. Prout: We haven't gotten any for quite some time because of the articles Dr. Martin pointed out which said there was nothing to it and just about clobbered any hope of funding.

Also the government has put out a flat rejection of any proposals of passing any current through the head including GSR. That's just pulled the rug out of any funding.

Audience member: How do you select subjects to be participants in this sort of thing?

Dr. Martin: We went through the files at our clinic and at Lancaster and pulled out people who looked like standard sensorineural hearing loss.

Audience member: What do you mean by standard hearing loss?

Dr. Martin: Standard sloping scores on puretones, standard scores on discrimination, moderate-severe SRT shifts from 20 - 80 dB. Pure tone thresholds from 10 - 90 dB.

Dr. Pratt: Have you ever been able to identify or isolate specific disorders, for example, known hair cell damage, known metabolic disorders or other types of problems where the therapy procedure seemed to be particularly efficient or more effective?

Dr. Martin: No. Once again it's too expensive in terms of time or money.

Dr. Pratt: Are you assuming in your experimental procedure that you do not have subjects with fluctuating hearing loss? If so, how would you select out subjects who presumably have fluctuating hearing loss from your population?

Dr. Martin: No, I don't think we assumed that at all. I'm sure that some of our patients had fluctuating hearing loss.

Dr. Studebaker: Your point is well taken about the very significant effect of the negative articles, particularly the one by Blair Simmons. My question is you have raised some questions regarding the procedures and results of Dr. Simmons and Dr. Glattke in this study. Have you contacted them to ask for specific explanations regarding the problems you encountered in evaluating their work?

Dr. Martin: I have attempted to contact them but have not been successful. Which means of course that I haven't tried very hard. Okay?

Dr. Pratt: One of the problems we face in the medical world

is research done by people who really aren't researchers. And perhaps that might be why the problems we're having now really might be relative to the fundamental basic research involved and why there were some wrong statements made. Do you think that's a possibility, that if you contacted them that there may be some retractions and you could continue your research or not?

Dr. Martin: My own view is that this is a well-known phenomenon called the Rosenthal effect in psychology. Rosenthal has made a career of examining people's mistakes. When the results come out in the way you expect you never check what you've done. When the results come out in the way you didn't expect you go back and check. It's possible that just because you expect certain results, just because your student thinks you expect certain results, when you get certain results you just don't bother to double check and I expect that's just what happened.

Dr. Pratt: I think that's a valid point that there are so few really good researchers.

Dr. Martin: I don't think it has to do with competency of researchers.

Dr. Pratt: Oh, I think so because there are many people .. ... I lived through the grant period of where I was held back in the medical academic world because I didn't do research and grants. Well most people really didn't do research, they just took a grant and played around with some animals and wrote a paper.

Dr. Martin: I would never accuse.......

Dr. Pratt: I think we have to become more observant of the medical literature. We always have statements coming out from paper to another relative to "so and so said this", but I found that this is acceptable. Do you feel that these other papers have repressed your research?

Dr. Martin: I'm not concerned with this. I'm just concerned with discovering the truth. I think that there were significant errors in the Glattke and Simmons papers. There are errors in procedure and design and in reporting the data. However, I'm not a conspiracy theorist and I think it just a matter of continuing to do work and getting it out at meetings like this.

Dr. Millin: I think from a clinical point of view something like this should be expanded and I'd like to see other people do the research and it's sad if our research efforts were suppressed especially now with money problems. This seems to have some validity and clinical potential and I personally would like to see it continued.

Mr. Yanick: I'd definitely like to see more research done and I'd like to see the groups that are tested screened for fluctuant hearing loss. There's a possibility that discrimination may be fluctuating and/or pure tones may be fluctuating. I think they should be carefully screened because fluctuating hearing loss is a common occurrence, although it's not realized to be common by the medical profession or by most audiologists. I think a series of audiograms should be done on people before they are admitted into a double-blind study.

Audience member: Did you investigate or examine the possibility of obtaining a medical-legal waiver? A signing away of the right of holding the experimenter responsible for effects of the therapy?

Dr. Martin: We had them do that but we knew it wouldn't make any difference. Legally it wouldn't make any difference at all because the patient could say he didn't understand it.

I would also like to point out that it's true in many cases that we have fluctuating hearing losses. Those kinds of fluctuations are probably not responsible for the changes we found because we were doing studies on groups of subjects and we are using controls and we would expect that the control subjects would be just as likely to have fluctuating losses as do the experimental subjects. Therefore, I feel the question is important but not essential to the question of if the therapy works.